Fast Forwards

UNLEASHING RESERVES OF WILLPOWER YOU NEVER KNEW YOU HAD

NOEL LYONS, MSc

Published By WellCoach UK

ISBN: 9798393405601

Praise for 'Fast Forwards'

"This succinct round-up of the science might surprise you. Helps explain how willpower, despite being at times somewhat intangible and polarizing, is something everyone can tap into and harness once they better understand how it really works."

- Nick Webster. Account Executive / Oxford University Alumnus.

"A thought provoking lively insight into the power of the human mind and our desire to aspire to be better at the "things" we love whilst allowing us to believe it is ok to let go of those "things" that inherently hold us back. I thoroughly enjoyed reading it and found myself nodding in a lot of places. It came along at the right time!"

- Sarah McDonald. Team GB Age Group Triathlete (50-55).

"This book offers a comprehensible approach for maximising one's potential in all areas of life. Loved the punchy paragraphs - made it easier to stay focused on the message rather than getting lost in blocks of text. Knowing Noel on a personal level too, the philosophies demonstrated in this book are clear to see. Noel is one of the most driven athletes that I have ever met."

- Cameron Payas. Accountant and 3.52 min 1500m Runner.

ACKNOWLEDGMENTS

My philosophy on willpower has been influenced by reading and listening to Roy Baumeister, the American social psychologist, and Kelly McGonigal, the health psychologist. Thank you both.

I would also like to thank all the scientific researchers mentioned in Further Reading for all their hard work and valuable insights too.

"No matter what you achieve, somebody helps you.
Behind the creation that we call our own are the thoughts and efforts of many."
- Althea Gibson

CONTENTS

1. INTRODUCTION

As a coach, allow me to begin by posing you the quintessential willpower question:

> Who would you BE
> What type of life would you HAVE
> If you could DO... what needed to be done
> (whether you felt like it or not)?

I admit to being a fan of all things drive, determination, grit, and mental toughness, including willpower. Not only have I read countless articles and books in this area, but I've also spent over 40 years as a competitive athlete myself and led quite a colourful and adventurous life by many people's standards.

I've also witnessed the rich and exciting lives certain other people live - the ones who make things happen. They lead successful professional lives and still find time to excel in sports or physical hobbies. They enjoy above-average health, rewarding social relationships, and uplift others around them etc.

There's a quote by Timothy Pychyl, a former university professor, 'When we procrastinate on our goals, we are basically putting off our lives.' I take this to mean, there's the life we are living... and then there's the life we could be living - if we stopped letting our mood, certain people, and unsettling events etc. get in our way. That's why willpower matters.

I guess that's why I felt compelled to write this book. On the one hand, I'm only too aware of the compounding value of willpower across a lifetime. Yet I also know it's not an attribute most people readily identify with. Plus, willpower has gotten a bad rap of late, with work-life balance and burnout becoming increasingly hot topics.

Well, what if the nature of willpower was not quite as simple, 'black-and-white', or 'either-or' as some would have you believe. What if there was a bigger picture to take in. Would you be interested in finding out more?

I hope so! Because your ability to persevere towards future goals with, ideally, passion and grace, is an important part of the success equation in life. In contrast, not feeling up to taking on new projects or seeing your goals through to completion can result in stress, low self-worth, and a general blah feeling towards life.

Be that as it may, I would also like to emphasise that there's a healthy balance to be found between striving hard and recharging yourself. So rest assured, I'm not going to ask you to become superhuman, just your truest, best self!

"Everyone has a vocation to be someone, but he (she) must understand clearly that in order to fulfil this vocation he (she) can only be one person: Himself (Herself)." - Thomas Merton.

Is Strong Willpower an Unrealistic Expectation?

Willpower continues to divide popular opinion perhaps because it is complex in so many ways. Even among academics, there is no generally accepted theory of willpower. Instead, there are many fascinating observations from a variety of diverse perspectives, different disciplines, and fields of inquiry. Whilst promising premises have been debated and nuances noted, there is no recognised model or framework necessary to bring about a consensus agreement.

It's precisely why I would like to invite you to keep an open mind in the chapters ahead. To consider what might be some new or novel perspectives around willpower that could benefit you, or at least change your current attitude towards willpower for the better.

There's also one overarching theme in this book, which, if you grasp it, could make all the difference between you *forcefully striving* or *effortlessly thriving* your way through life.

To make such an audacious claim, I have dug deep into the psychology and science behind willpower. So rest assured, what follows is not just my opinion. Nor am I merely attempting to appeal to whatever is popular, mainstream, or trending right now. It's scientifically informed and further directed by my extensive real-world expertise. All research papers consulted are thereby included in Further Reading under their relevant chapter categories. However, I've also refrained from making this an academic piece of writing, as my target audience simply wants to see willpower demystified.

"Complex" need not equate to "complicated." Everything can be made simpler, although please do not expect a simple, generic solution to willpower that works under all circumstances. Life does not come with an instruction manual. Instead everyone was gifted with a more than adequate brain. With this in mind, each chapter in this book will present key findings and principles surrounding willpower that you can integrate into your thinking today.

WHY LISTEN TO ME?

I promise to keep this brief, and you are welcome to skip over this section. It's just that some people like a little background information.

Here it is. I've been extremely fortunate at times in my life to coach professionally, and mix personally, with some highly successful and even mega-wealthy people. Their influence has rubbed off on me, especially the world-class sports stars and how they arrived there. My own background is modest, although as a disclaimer, I did go to a grammar school. Yet throughout my life, I have always challenged myself to grow and evolve, whether that be through travel (overseas work experience around the world); academically (Birmingham and Bristol University); or sport (Kent county runner, triathlon elite race license and GB age-group including Ironman).

All of which has provided me with a better understanding of willpower than if I had just researched it, read about it, or watched a bunch of YouTube videos. Add to that over thirty years of assisting clients in making positive lifestyle changes.

As a result, rather than adopting a blind faith or dogmatic belief in the science alone, it has given me a practical bias and an intuitive sense for what works. A big difference-maker given there's such a wealth of research papers on willpower and other closely related areas like self-control, self-regulation, self-discipline, etc.

Indeed, it's rewarding to see that a large part of my success now - as an executive coach - comes from empowering clients to stretch far beyond what they thought was possible, when they first started working with me.

WHO STANDS TO BENEFIT FROM THIS BOOK?

Perhaps:

You've been feeling your energy, vitality, and enthusiasm waning of late.

You want to raise your game, and take your mindset to the next level.

You've been feeling more confused, overrun, and exhausted recently.

You want to break a cycle of setting goals and giving up soon after.

The stresses of daily life are messing with your health and fitness levels.

You're intrigued and eager to learn more about the latest psychology behind willpower, self-discovery, and how your brain works.

Finally, if you're feeling stuck or finding it difficult to get started with a million things on your plate.

Specifically, I think you can gain from this book if you are in any way ambitious and have found yourself spinning your wheels. Our goals and aspirations often prove more challenging and take longer to achieve than when first conceived. That restless agitated feeling is often your mind intelligently signaling your body that you're ready to make some important changes!

The answer is not always about taking smaller steps or down-sizing your expectations. Sometimes it has more to do with expanding and/or reframing your mindset. The return being that with greater momentum and fulfilment in life comes more motivation and energy. Isn't that what you've been lacking lately?

WHAT CAN YOU EXPECT TO LEARN?

This guidebook is made up of three main parts.

The first part (chapter one) addresses why willpower is necessary and how it works.

The second part (chapters two to six) examines the five key components that influence willpower.

The final part (chapter seven) attempts to put theory into practise by providing a workable framework for unleashing - previously hidden - reserves of willpower.

My promise: Once you comprehend how the various pieces of the willpower puzzle fit together, you'll be armed with all the conviction you need to navigate your chosen path in life.

Steering yourself in the direction of your 'best' self' will also lead to greater personal satisfaction and well-being. Yes, it's possible to find fulfilment right where you are, without quitting your job or making huge life changes.

Discover too how to celebrate living more courageously, replacing passivity with boldness, and how to stay on track without feeling forced to constantly push yourself. In the process, learn to banish imposter syndrome and overconfidence for good.

As ever, my emphasis will be on offering you actionable insights derived from mixing research-based wisdom with practical expertise.

Are you ready? I hope so. Let's get you started then. After all, haven't you been putting off your life long enough?!

Coaching Reflection Questions:

Nobody can give you wiser advice than yourself. So ask yourself:

- Why don't you always do... what you know you should do?

- Why do you feel unstoppable some days… and easily deflatable on others?

- How much are you relying on willpower to propel you through each day?

- How often do you cave in to impulses or cravings?

- How often do you self-distract with your phone?

- How often do you numb your feelings with food?

- How many poor decisions do you think you make due to weak willpower?

- What might be possible for you if you became more self-disciplined?

- What if you could make smarter decisions - more often?

- What if you were able to focus better, for longer periods of time?

- Compound all of this over months or years, what might be possible then?

- Would that make reading and digesting this entire book worthwhile?!

"Always do your best.
What you plant now, you will harvest later."
- Og Mandino

2. THE AKRASIA EFFECT

In its simplest form, willpower is the ability to say NO. It's the power that enables you to resist a temptation, in order to attain a more desirable outcome later.

We often exert willpower alongside closely related personal characteristics, such as determination, drive, decisiveness, restraint, resolve, grit, self-regulation, self-discipline, and self-control.

No surprise then that those individuals with high willpower largely fare better in life across most areas: health (physical, mental, and emotional), happiness, wealth, relationships, success, overcoming adversity… etc.

The reverse is also true. There's good evidence that low willpower levels represent a collective concern within communities:

"Most major problems, personal and social, centre on failure of self-control: compulsive spending and borrowing, impulsive violence, underachievement in school, procrastination at work, alcohol and drug abuse, unhealthy diet, lack of exercise, chronic anxiety, and explosive anger." - Roy Baumeister + John Tierney.

With that said, if you perceive yourself as lacking in willpower, relax!

Willpower is certainly a desirable quality to possess, yet few people rank themselves highly on it. According to the VIA institute, only 5% possess "self-regulation" as a major strength.

No wonder then, many people feel as if they are in a perennial battle with themselves, even when they resolve to act differently in the future.

It's not just modern-times either, but centuries-old. 'Akrasia' is the word used by the ancient Greeks to describe 'the state of mind in which someone acts against their better judgement, through weakness of will.'

Positive expectation helps, but alone is not enough. The brain is a poor appraiser of future rewards, both overestimating and underestimating how good it will feel to reach any goal. It's also biased, prioritising guaranteed rewards over delayed rewards. As a result, it's predisposed to settle for an immediate reward (i.e. the easier and more obvious option), than wait for a potentially better future reward. As Baylor Barbee once said, 'free cheese is always available in mousetraps!' Here I recommend the paper on desire and rewards by Dobryakova and Smith (2022) in Further Reading.

Neurobiology also teaches us there's a clash between the two systems that play key roles in decision-making. A reactive system in the amygdala (limbic area of the brain) that assesses the pros and cons of an immediate reward - that clashes with a reflective system (in the prefrontal cortex or PFC) that does the same for future rewards.

The two systems assess whether the level of effort is worthwhile in view of the costs and benefits associated with achievement of the goal. Essentially, an internal conflict between two appealing options: instant gratification or long-term satisfaction. The result: uncertainty, which inclines our brain to make sub-optimal decisions or helplessly dither.

Walter Mischel dubbed it the "Hot-Cool" System:

Hot = simple, fast; but also driven by emotions and impulse.
Cool = rational, thinking part (making informed, reflective decisions).

The hot system develops early in life, whereas the cool system is much later (i.e. mid-to-late twenties). Ever wondered why some teenagers take silly risks?!

"Do not pray for easy lives, pray to be stronger men." - John F. Kennedy.

Another factor to consider is that we all have a tendency to think that we will have more willpower, energy, time, and motivation tomorrow. We convince ourselves that our future self will somehow be an upgrade to our current self. The snag being, that presented with the opportunity to make a different choice tomorrow, we almost always 'give in' to temptation today. When our long-term goals have less urgency, it's easy to keep putting things off for some day. Soon 'not trying' or 'quitting easily' becomes the norm, with negative consequences.

Add on recurrent demands without sufficient recovery, and it paves the way for sub-optimal lifestyle choices, which further spark poor lifestyle habits. Feeling tired and wired is now normal. We avoid challenges. We become easily emotionally charged to everyday triggers. Lapses become commonplace. We can languish or, worse, drift in-and-out of struggle mode. All part of a vicious cycle that hinders subsequent willpower attempts.

Before long, we deem the thought of mobilising willpower as impossible, or too costly and tiring. When we expect fatigue, we exert less effort and for less time. A lack of willpower then becomes self-fulfilling, since beliefs beget behaviours.

It can prove hard to break free from this kind of self-perpetuating loop: low energy - little interest – a lack of motivation - feelings of passivity, pointlessness, or hopelessness – avoidance of decision making - maladaptive response patterns (impulsivity, rumination) - less likely to seize the initiative, etc. All of which, interestingly, are presenting conditions for 'mental health' disorders!

In addition, repeatedly testing your willpower causes your brain to function differently. Not only is it harder to refrain from the usual temptations without adequate recovery or regeneration, but you also feel the same urges more strongly. It's why it's that much harder to muster up willpower, when you're already feeling down or overloaded.

With all this in mind, is it not reasonable to assume we are all doomed to the Akrasia Effect?! Is relying on willpower not futile?

Here is what is important to remember:

There are other factors which influence individual willpower - over and above the brain itself.

Yes, the nature of willpower is complex, with many compounding variables, which rules out an effortless miracle solution or simple hacks. However, it is possible to tease out some key principles and ways of framing willpower - in order to more effectively benefit from this prized inner strength.

Are you ready to start in strengthening your willpower?

Chapter two reveals the crucial, supportive role biology plays in providing the foundational structure for willpower.

KEY CHAPTER TAKEAWAYS:

- The better you understand how your brain works, the better you can understand yourself (and others). Advances in neurobiology can assist us with this.

- Willpower extends beyond just saying NO. It also calls for aligning one's actions, with personal values and aspirations in the face of inner motivational conflicts.

- Willpower is a brain attribute, not a personality gift (that some have - others don't). Everyone possesses the capability to better manage this inner strength and to build greater reserves.

3. WILLPOWER IS PART WELL POWER

"Willpower is as much how you fuel - as how you feel."

Wellpower is synonymous with your sense of vibrancy.

It's also perhaps the most ignored route to more willpower.

Many individuals now understand the advantages of a good diet, quality sleep, regular physical activity, mindfulness, meditation, and stress reduction, etc. However, the power of each discipline multiplies when applied collectively, and where allowed to compound with time.

That said, there is no standard 'wellpower' prescription that works for everyone. Each one of us must determine for ourselves which preferences fit best with our personal commitments, and which bring out our highest self the most often.

Breaking it down further, it would take an entire book to do justice to all that contributes to wellpower. The purpose of what follows is merely to support and reinforce the central thrust of this chapter. Namely, that willpower is as much how you fuel as it is how you feel.

SLEEP
"Your future depends on your dreams, so go to sleep." – Mesut
Barazany.

Sleep is the number one recovery tool. Hence, the cliché phrase: 'Just sleep on it.'

Sleep deprivation deactivates neuroplasticity, stunting learning and growth. It causes us to become more susceptible to cravings and temptations, makes controlling emotions and focusing attention more difficult, and leads us to over-react to stressors.

Just one night of sleep deprivation is all it takes to impair our brain's ability to filter out irrelevant information, thus making it more distractible. We make it worse still, when we allow sleep debt to accumulate.

The prefrontal cortex (PFC) is especially hard hit, affecting impulse control, decision-making and memory. Left unchecked, it can lead to impulse control and attention problems similar to hyperactivity and attention deficit disorder. All of which is bad news for willpower. No wonder we end up making bad choices when we skimp on sleep.

It's also easily remedied. When the sleep-deprived catch a better night's sleep, their brain scans no longer show signs of PFC impairment. A good night's sleep helps your brain and body manage energy better. It also re-establishes your default nature to be calm and alert when called upon.

So if you spot yourself yawning and/or under-performing each day, aim to get more quality sleep each night (ideally between six to eight hours).

It's worth checking out 'The Matt Walker Podcast' - which is all about sleep, the brain, and the body – if sleeping is an area you could improve in.

FOOD CHOICES
"Food is like a pharmaceutical compound that affects the brain." -
Fernando Gómez-Pinilla.

Willpower depletion has a biological basis, notably lower blood-glucose levels and decreased activity in the anterior cingulate cortex. All normal brain functions (e.g. thinking, learning, memory) depend on glucose.

This is where special glucose-detecting cells can determine whether your blood levels are increasing, decreasing or stable. If your brain detects declining amounts, it cuts back on energy-draining tasks like willpower.

This would explain why your willpower is weaker when you're hungry or dieting (i.e. your blood sugar is low). Also, why you might then find your willpower depleted in other, unrelated life challenges.

Surely it is far better to direct your willpower towards building healthy habits that last, than use it to fend off cravings? Strict diets alongside strenuous workouts only add to your overall stress levels and willpower demands - negatively impacting your health and happiness.

Low glucose levels also affect your body as much as your brain, contributing to a general sense of tiredness. So maintaining stable glucose levels is imperative for promoting general well-being and even ageing slower.

So, for some, rebooting run-down willpower could be as simple as restoring blood glucose levels to normal. The right nutrition can give you more energy, reduce cravings, and improve decision-making.

Best practise is to eat whole natural foods (at regular intervals) without added sugars, saturated fat or chemicals. Eating a substantial breakfast will provide your brain with energy at the start of the day. Try eating mindfully, slowing down, savouring your food, and appreciating each bite. This can help with portion control and with feeling less food-deprived. If you practise when alone, it will be easier for you when eating out with friends.

However, it's not just food. Many things impact on blood sugar levels. Factors like sleep, exercise, lean muscle mass, stress etc. which is why the right eating choices will help, but not as much as getting your entire lifestyle habits working together in harmony.

Try tracking and monitoring with a continuous glucose monitor (CGMs). If you are a metabolically compromised person (e.g. overweight, midsection body fat, or metabolic syndrome), it might just make a difference in helping you get a grip on food cravings throughout the day.

As for alcohol, it acts as an inhibitory neurotransmitter in the brain, significantly disrupting your sleep and subsequent performance. So limit alcohol to 1 or 2 drinks a week for optimal brain function.

Also, best restrict coffee to 1 to 2 cups, and mornings only, given that it can take up to 10-12 hours to clear caffeine completely from your bloodstream. In addition, stay hydrated with filtered water, as this too will enhance sleep quality, cognition, and mood.

EXERCISE / PHYSICAL ACTIVITY

'Just ten minutes of exercise had significantly altered their dopamine circuits and increased their willpower.' - Alex Korb.

Daily physical activity keeps your brain healthy, especially the Prefrontal Cortex (PFC). It also enhances your overall sense of well-being, with the release of a bunch of 'feel-good chemicals.'

The simple process of exercising leads to profound changes in the brain at any age. It doesn't take months of training either. As little as five minutes daily can contribute to building or restoring willpower.

So whilst you might think it takes willpower to exercise, exercise can improve willpower. As can most sports, skills and hobbies that involve challenging oneself through physical activity.

As Kelly McGonigal remarked, "I don't think it's a coincidence that many people are drawn to communities where they can pursue physical challenges alongside others."

Better still, regular physical activity can infuse new found strength into all areas of your life. This then gives you more willpower for when and where you need it most. This might mean better focus at work, less procrastination, feeling more in control of your emotions, or sticking to healthier lifestyle habits overall.

It's why exercise, diet and sleep are major 'keystone habits.'

Physical activity reduces stress and improves sleep quality. It might also buffer and offset the negative effects of stress, and a lack of sleep, with its mood-enhancing qualities. Have you yourself not experienced a more productive day all-round, when you made time for physical movement?

The reverse is also true. Willpower is rarely just an exercise or food problem. A lack of willpower will show up in all areas of your life in varying degrees.

Two plausible brain mechanisms may explain how exercise can strengthen willpower. Both relate to the promise of reward:

(a) a decrease in effort costs combined with a greater efficiency of brain regions involved in the task and/or (b) an increase in the value of effort within the context of high effort and high reward (i.e. an increase in motivation to exert effort). Please see Audiffren et al. (2022) in Further Reading.

Pathway (a) fits with what we know about how the brain experiences 'exercise' as a kind of stress. It adapts by increasing brain-derived neurotrophic factor (BDNF), a protein that supports the growth, survival and communication between neurons in the brain.

This builds the brain up to be both bigger (i.e. grey matter or brain cells) and faster (i.e. white matter or insulation on brain cells that help them communicate with each other). As a result, BDNF improves how networks in your brain use energy.

We also know BDNF increases long-term potentiation - a pattern of activity where new memory circuits get stimulated by new experiences - which might also benefit willpower in gauging future rewards?

MINDFULNESS

'Mindfulness is a way of befriending ourselves and our experience.' - Jon Kabat-Zinn

Mindfulness is a huge topic with many varied ways to practise it.

Here I just want to make a few general points relevant to willpower. Modern-lives are not simple. An increased array of choices can leave you feeling 'uncertain', or constantly looking to better yourself. Add in sleep deprivation, small children, elderly parents, demanding job or work colleagues etc. and the demands multiply. The more overwhelmed you feel, the more you may gain from gaining greater clarity about yourself. Especially when the tendencies of people who struggle with willpower are poor self-knowledge, reactive by nature, and easily distracted.

Now here's the proviso - find a way of practising mindfulness that works for you. For me, it's an active form like running or cycling outdoors because I can't sit still for long without a good enough reason. It becomes valuable thinking time as well as a chance to relieve any tension pent up that day.

The principal goal is deeper self-awareness. Not about becoming someone better, but befriending who you already are. To better understand our own wiring, and bodily sensations.

It's not about thinking you're weak, flawed, or feeling obliged to change how you are feeling. It's about nurturing the relationship between your current self and future self.

It's through self-awareness that we foster self-acceptance and permission to be our most authentic selves (i.e. pursuing the values and goals meaningful personally to us).

In doing so, we gain valuable psychological distancing from our ego, allowing us to reconstruct our internal mental representations (e.g. thoughts / images / memories) in adaptive ways.

You could also simply choose to reflect on past events, or contemplate interesting concepts, if that appeals to you more.

As for the biological effects of mindfulness on brain function, the research is still in the early stages. However, indications are that mindfulness can alter the brain in a variety of ways.

These include:

- Increasing grey matter density (pivotal in processing information and perspective forming).
- Changing brain waves (increasing alpha and theta brain waves, which are associated with relaxation and introspection)
- Decreasing amygdala activity (helping to reduce stress and improve emotional regulation).
- Increasing functional connectivity (especially involved in attention and emotion regulation).
- Modulating pain perception (by altering activity in brain regions involved in the processing of pain).

The parts of the brain believed to be implicated include:

- Prefrontal cortex (increasing grey matter density and blood flow)
- Amygdala (dialing down activity)
- Insula (increasing awareness of one's own emotions and physical sensations)
- Hippocampus (increases grey matter density, related to improved contextual learning and visual-spatial memory)
- Anterior cingulate cortex (involved in attention and emotion regulation, linking with other brain regions).

Such changes may be seen within just 6-8 weeks of brief, regular practise. It follows then that improvements in multiple areas such as emotion regulation, stress reduction, and increased focus and attention (i.e. as a result of mindfulness practise), might also contribute to strengthening willpower.

In addition, given the similarities between the biological benefits of exercise and mindfulness, that combining them both would likely be even more powerful?

"Exercise alone provides psychological and physical benefits. However, if you also adopt a strategy that engages your mind while you exercise, the effect is often stronger and even quicker" - James Rippe M.D.

MEDITATION

"The quieter you become, the more you can hear." - Ram Dass

If you don't feel comfortable with your own thoughts or silence, meditation is another option for improving the biological basis of willpower.

Personally, I am not a fan of guided meditations or a guru 'directing my thoughts.' However, I do frequently use focus music, biannual beats and similar. I find they calm my mind and help counter against constant stimulation, plus reduce external distractions.

The important thing with meditation - just like mindfulness - is just to be with it. The goal is not to become a master meditator, but to master you better. So stay patient. Don't judge it. When you don't feel like it, do it anyway.

It's natural that some days will prove harder than others. Remember, being "bad" at it - constantly pushing away intrusive thoughts or staying with unpleasant sensations that are arising - is also what trains your brain to act with better self-control.

Finally, practice often. Consistency outperforms duration. The more you do, the greater the overall lasting effects.

As for its effects, meditation is known to activate some regions of the brain and deactivate others.

For instance, it dials up the Prefrontal Cortex (involved in thinking) and the Hypothalamus (which connects with other brain areas).

Conversely, it dials down the Parietal Lobes (which can lessen our sense of self) and the amygdala (involved in emotional regulation). All of which helps improve overall brain function.

Plus, by lowering stress and levels of cortisol in the body, it can help reshape the gut/brain axis connection for the better.

NATURE

"There are benefits of spending time in nature (and leaving technology behind) such as improved short-term memory, enhanced working memory, better problem-solving, greater creativity, lower levels of stress and higher feelings of positive well-being." David Strayer.

A simple five-minute walk or run outside in nature can reduce your stress levels, boost your mood, and help replenish your willpower reserves. Regular activity is better still - ideally in a mindful or observational state - in whatever outdoor location is most appealing or convenient: Green woodlands/park/field, blue sea/river, or white snow space. Make it a habit of stepping away from everyday responsibilities to refresh, or even totally reboot if need be.

Research also points towards significant improvement in working memory after nature walks —up to 20% - which leads to improved impulse control.

STRESS

"It isn't the mountain ahead that wears you out; it's the grain of sand in your shoe." — Robert Service

The negative side of stress is that it interrupts our thoughts in the moment leaving us to act instinctively and impulsively. It shifts your brain into a reward seeking state, encouraging you to zoom in on immediate, short-term outcomes. This is in contrast to willpower which requires you keeping the bigger picture in mind, so as to foresee the consequences of any action.

Further, under stress, the sympathetic system dominants. Your body is in a constantly mobilised state and is 'wasting energy'. Meanwhile, the parasympathetic is not being turned on enough, leading to insufficient recovery. After a while, it can feel 'normal.' Low levels of energy, willpower and health become accepted as inevitable consequences of modern-day living.

If left unaddressed, stress can impair our ability to operate efficiently in the long run. Long-term stress raises biochemical stress compounds in the body such as cortisol. These can trigger a loop of chronic stress, lack of sleep, poor choices and damage to your brain - causing distracted thoughts and overly emotional reactions.

We become more likely to be tempted and find ourselves 'losing control' more often. We shift towards self-preservation mode. Feeling better now or finding relief assumes greater importance than pursuing longer-term goals or making authentic choices (i.e. based on standards, values and commitments).

So much so, that we can soon find ourselves no longer motivated to take on long-term goals. Suffice to say, learning how to better manage your stress levels is one of the most important things you can do to boost your willpower!

Stress, though, is always the last piece of the well-being puzzle people wish to acknowledge or confront. Many try eating better, exercising more, meditating and/or sleeping well… etc. only to relapse. Yet in managing your stress levels well, you can better accommodate other healthy lifestyle practises. Hence, for many people living a high-tech and fast-paced lifestyle, stress relief should be a higher priority.

Many books have been written on stress relief, with strategies falling into any one of three categories:

1) Delete or remove the source of stress.
2) Reframe how you view that stressor.
3) Adopt various coping strategies (where you accept stress as a part of your life).

A fourth alternative is seeing stress as a positive force.

If you perceive stress to be bad, you will feel its negative consequences more.

Conversely, if you can see the beneficial aspects of stress (e.g. it sharpens decision making, balances the immune system, and enhances alertness), you will experience it better.

You can reframe the same stressors to approach them in an alternative light - as interesting, exciting, different or challenging - awakening inner personal qualities, currently lying untested.

As I'm fond of telling clients: If you can't decrease your life demands, then look at raising your personal capacity. In this way, low-to-moderate levels of stress can help you grow and develop as a person.

REGENERATIVE BREAKS
"Just because you take breaks doesn't mean you're broken." — Curtis Jones

After a day of working hard on difficult cognitive tasks, glutamate accumulates in the forebrain. It's your brain's way of slowing down to manage the strain, similar to how lactate build-up in muscles during physical exercise protects against over-exertion.

Glutamate is the most abundant neurotransmitter in the brain, involved in multiple important networking brain functions. These include learning, memory, and decision-making. In addition, glutamate helps regulate energy metabolism in the brain, providing the energy needed for neurons to perform their functions. It also plays a role in the metabolism of glucose, the brain's primary source of energy.

Repeated cognitive demands lead to mental fatigue, especially blocks of deep work, since the brain has to repeatedly resist the appeal of doing something else less taxing. This fatigue is linked to recycling of the glutamate that builds-up during neural activity.

By ensuring "willpower renewal", through proper rest, relaxation and quality sleep, you'll face each day feeling replenished.

Regenerative breaks (aka strategic resting) should play a major part in your daily routine, with the key distinction being 'regenerative'. Some of the most common relaxation strategies are also the least effective ones: surfing the internet, social media scrolling, playing video games, and watching TV or movies (for more than 2 hours a day).

Whereas some of the most effective stress-relief strategies are:

Exercising/playing sports; praying, religious services or spiritual practices; reading; listening to music; spending time with friends or family; massages; meditation/yoga; outdoors in nature (fresh air + sunlight) and creative hobbies.

The advantage the more effective strategies have is that they also help us feel better. They boost mood-enhancing brain chemicals like serotonin, gamma-aminobutyric acid (GABA) and oxytocin. They also help shut down the brain's stress response, reduce stress hormones in the body, and induce the healing relaxation response.

So make time for fun things you enjoy and recharging recreational activities outside of work. Plan regular weekends or weeks away. View them as non-negotiables and investments.

Schedule regular check-ins with yourself to evaluate how you're feeling regarding your current physical, mental and emotional state. Rate your level of exhaustion or degree of life satisfaction.

Nurture meaningful inter-personal relationships. Connection and support can provide added resilience when life's inevitable challenges arise. Your mind and body – perhaps even your family - will thank you!

Low willpower levels may not be a case of working too hard, but of insufficient rest and recovery in-between. One of the reasons poor lifestyle habits arise in the first place is because we haven't built in enough social, fun, or pleasure time into our days. We may consider ourselves lazy and unmotivated; when the reality is we're contributing to burnout!

IN SUMMARY
"It's not that we have nasty impulses; our usual restraints are weakened."
– Roy Baumeister

Clearly, willpower has a biological basis.

Willpower requires executive or prefrontal cortex function. Executive or PFC function depends on wellpower. Both our brain and body need to be supported by the right environment. How well we sleep or eat, how far we move, how stressed we feel, etc. all nurture our overall mind-body connection. You give your best when you feel your best.

That said, I am not suggesting that high well-being is the solution to low willpower. More that it is a big part of the overall puzzle-piece, which often gets neglected.

If you regularly find yourself expending too much willpower, or are unable to fully replenish what gets expended each day, then a few simple tweaks in your weekly repertoire could make a real difference.

Intuitively, you already know this. Ask yourself now: When you are having a good day, what wellpower practise(s) do you have in place? Chances are you can tick off the boxes: Sleep - nutrition - physical activity - mindfulness/meditation - nature - regenerative breaks - music - connection with friends and family - low stress levels.

Digging further, which one is most pivotal for you? That is, the one(s) that sets you up for the entire day. For some, it might be a good night's sleep. For others, maybe an early morning workout, meditation, Yoga/Pilates session, or a balanced breakfast. It will vary from person to person.

For me, I ensure I sleep soundly each night. Exercising is also non-negotiable. Regardless of daily events, it will happen in some form. Another non-negotiable is my nutritional requirements, followed by regular regenerative breaks throughout the day. It's what you would expect from someone who values fitness and well-being amongst their top three values. See what works best for you and be prepared to experiment with different times of the day.

It strikes me that if willpower levels are down in society today, then it's no coincidence that well power levels are too.

What if instead we aimed to address life's demands like competitive athletes organise their weekly schedules? By constructing a lifestyle that supports our main goals, our personal commitments, and that takes into account: Exercising, eating, resting/relaxing, meditating, visualising, and sleeping/recovering.

We are all better prepared to take on willpower challenges when well-rested, well -nourished, well-slept, and not under undue stress.

It would reflect back to us in terms of increased productivity, mental and physical health, better relationships and life satisfaction. In short, we get to release our best self into the world, rather than as Henry Thoreau put it: 'live a life of quiet desperation.'

KEY CHAPTER TAKEAWAYS:

Willpower has a biological basis. Fuel your willpower engine. Please see André and Baumeister (2022) in Further Reading.

Willpower does not fail you. You sabotage it through low Wellpower levels. Willpower is as much how you fuel as how you feel.

Who are you at your BEST? Which lifestyle habits - in particular - help support this?

4 WILLPOWER IS PART WHO POWER

ARE YOU WITH OR WITHOUT WILLPOWER?

Do you see willpower as limited or unlimited? It's well-known: If you believe you have little willpower, then you are probably right.

Seeing willpower as limited becomes self-fulfilling. You hold back, don't try, or are quicker to quit when obstacles appear.

Similarly, if you believe that others have more willpower than you, you are less likely to stretch yourself.

It's rarely all or nothing. I've witnessed clients who can be strong concerning business matters but weak-willed, sticking to positive health and fitness habits. Once they recognise this, they can use that same determination in business to push through any discomfort when working-out.

The difference being then, seeing willpower as a state of mind you can shift into, as and when required.

This principle also works in reverse. Viewing willpower as an unlimited resource might just give you added motivation when needed.

Fatigue is signalled by an overprotective brain (that monitors body energy to prevent exhaustion). Hence, tiredness can be deceptive.

Once you realise this, you can summon additional motivation to push past perceived limits or to atone for feeling depleted. See Hoffer & Giddings (Oct 2015) in Further Reading.

ARE YOU CLEAR ON YOUR VALUES?

How clear are you in your top three or five core values? People can often rattle off multiple changes they want to make, without being clear on their underlying 'main thing' in life. This can lead to stress, overwhelm, and frustration. No wonder values are often the first subject life coaches tackle with clients.

I quote Angela Duckworth, a professor of psychology and expert on grit and self-control, 'nobody has passion and perseverance unless what they do aligns with their values.' Luciano Pavarotti, the opera singer, also said, 'people think I'm disciplined. It's not discipline. It's devotion. There's a great difference.'

Values are the neurological passions that drive you toward rewarding goals. They illustrate your priorities - shaped over time through experience - which become your memories and personal story (i.e. your sense of who you are).

Your values accordingly steer your choices and enable you to recover quicker from setbacks. Each time you affirm a core personal value to yourself; you reinforce its value, and shore up your sense of self-worth.

In fact, the clearer you know and the stronger you cherish your values, the easier it will be for you to summon willpower in order to honour them. Best, you will likely feel energised doing so, as value-affirming evokes psychological well-being. See Schmeichel and Vohs (2009) in Further Reading.

By becoming more intentional in your actions - through vision or action boards - you strengthen the hot emotional 'wants' system as referred to in chapter one. Otherwise your brain gives it lower priority, relative to your cool rational system (which prioritises necessities like paying your bills and keeping you psychologically safe).

Thus, daily visualisations, affirmations, and savouring practises provide life with meaning and direction - as well as kindling reserves of willpower for when you need them.

ARE YOU CLEAR ON YOUR PERSONAL STANDARDS?

Our Personal Standards are the bright lines by which we choose to live, governing what we are prepared to tolerate, and dovetailing with willpower in their maintenance. First, the standards of desirable behaviour get set. Then you need both the motivation to meet them and the ability to monitor them via heightened awareness (of circumstances and actions).

So think… how can you shape your everyday actions to better uphold the values and personal standards you identify most with? Because as William Somerset Maugham is often quoted, 'it's a funny thing about life; if you refuse to accept anything but the best, you very often get it.'

HOW CONSCIENTIOUSNESS ARE YOU?

What tracking tools are you using to help you navigate through life? 'Conscientiousness' is one of the big five personality traits. Out of all of them, it is the one most closely linked to higher levels of willpower levels. It helps individuals to shape both their environment and daily behaviour patterns.

'Organised' people are renown for committing to multiple positive habits. As a result, "conscientious" people usually look biologically younger, walk faster and experience better lifelong health. Here apps, checklists, and scoreboards might help you cultivate this personality trait.

HOW STRONG ARE YOUR RELIGIOUS BELIEFS?

Religion clearly defines standards of behaviour. Plus, we know prayer and meditation directly impact the part of the human brain responsible for willpower and decision-making. This might explain why religious people have more willpower than average and are often better at achieving their aspirations. Or maybe it's the eventuality of being under observation by a higher power that helps to keep that person's actions in check? Also, when a person considers a goal to be 'holy' or 'sacred,' they will put more effort into achieving it.

HOW STRONG (AND HOW OFTEN) DO YOU EXPERIENCE POSITIVE EMOTIONS?

Is willpower all about good reason, logic, and analysis? Not according to the work of David DeSteno - a professor of psychology - who has studied emotional strategies.

We know that people who struggle most with willpower are often in a chronic state of tension or high stress. Compare with positive emotions, which by their very nature, equate to a less stressed state. However, David suggests it's less about happiness per se, and more about these three specific states: compassion (for self and for others); gratitude and pride.

Just like willpower, they are personal qualities you can grow and nurture. Yet what's extra-special about these three is that they also qualify as co-operative, adaptive or pro-social emotions. Displaying them regularly might act like a booster shot for willpower, helping us become more patient and future-orientated in our choices. Knowing this, an individual could leverage them to invest in their own best future self.

Cultivating Compassion

Blaming or criticising yourself weakens willpower. Yes, holding high personal standards helps tease the best out of us. However, we also need to remain kind to ourselves when we fall short of our own expectations, as guaranteed we will.

Everybody experiences setbacks or makes mistakes. We all face frequent disappointments and feelings of frustration with slow progress. What's more pertinent is how we handle them. It's prudent to expect difficulties. Think too how might a supportive friend or coach respond - someone who believes in you, and wants only the best for you? Your attitude towards challenges, and towards yourself, is pivotal to you in making continued progress.

People who experience shame or guilt are more likely to relapse than those who cut themselves some slack. Regret increases stress and shifts our brains into a reward-seeking state. This pushes us back towards the very thing we feel bad about because that behaviour is our crutch. Think dieters who break their diet and then turn to comfort food. Soon we can find ourselves in a downward spiral, no longer in control.

However, people with high willpower accept and integrate their competing selves. So be mindful of your feelings. Forgive yourself. Normalise any feelings of guilt and shame.

Recognise that failures and setbacks are part of life. They are rarely terminal. It only takes five minutes to break the cycle.

Five minutes… of exercise and you are back on track.
Five minutes… of writing and your book is moving forward again.
Five minutes… to feel good about yourself again.

Saying all this, it's important to state that self-forgiveness alone is not enough. Your real freedom lies in your choices. So accept responsibility. Take an objective stance. What situational factors were at play? Could you have acted differently? How might you respond?

Self-reflection and a willingness to change are the leading drivers of change. Punish yourself and you miss out on learning how to succeed the next time!

There's also an unexpected benefit. Compassion for others starts with self-compassion. Those capable of showing self-compassion are more likely to show compassion to other people.

Our own vulnerabilities and failings don't make us weak. They enable us to feel greater empathy towards other people. Those just like us, who find themselves in a similar position. It's this shared sense of connection that can help motivate you to care about others, without having previously received any benefits from them in return.

In addition, framing our choices based on how they affect others can also help us make wiser choices for ourselves.

Growing Gratitude

Feeling grateful, more often, helps reduce impulsive behaviours. But the true power of gratitude lies not just in its expression. It comes from its shaping of behaviour and appraising situations in ways that allow you to appreciate other people's efforts, support, and kindness.

For example, grateful people are more patient in the moment, as well as more ready to invest in their future self, which encourages perseverance.

Finally, gratitude boosts dopamine and serotonin, which contribute to your well-being. Take ten minutes each day to record ten things you are grateful for. Bonus points awarded if you can then express and share your gratitude with someone else.

Protecting Pride

Authentic pride is a pride that stems from proven possession of a valued ability. This pushes you to persevere in the face of difficulty in acquiring skills that will benefit you in the long run. But for pride to work, we must pair it with humility. That no matter your skill set, each of us depends on each other, requiring willingness to give and take.

We can then leverage pride by working on skills those around you value; by keeping a journal that tracks your success, your aspirations and your progress (not always a linear trajectory!) and giving meaningful, effort-based praise to others.

Emotional Intelligence

Finally, higher levels of 'emotional intelligence' result in less procrastination. See Eckert (2016) in Further Reading.

It would seem that the better able we are to understand and address our own emotions, alongside those of other people; the better able we are to make sense of our environment and adjust to it accordingly (in pursuit of our goals).

HOW WELL DO YOU IDENTIFY WITH YOUR 'FUTURE SELF'?

'Strong willpower extends beyond strong will.'

Metaphorically speaking, we have one brain shared by two minds: 'Default You' and 'Aspirational You.'

Default you is less about you, and more about societal programming, favouring comfort and instant gratification. The concern is, when we settle for what's most convenient, we are in effect trading the satisfaction of success for not feeling disappointed. It's also human nature to kid ourselves that if something isn't available to us, then we don't really want it. We do it to protect ourselves; often based on our past rather than our current possibilities.

This may suit the moment, but longer-term every choice has consequences, even no choice at all. It reminds me of Grandmother Janou's remark in the 1939 film 'Love Affair': 'Life will one day present you with the tab' (referring to Charles Boyer's character, Michel). The decisions we make compound throughout life, eventually catching up with us. It's why it's vital to reawaken 'Aspirational You' - that part of you which aspires to a brighter future.

This illustrates why strong willpower extends beyond strong will. It also demands the wisdom to pursue what's in your best interest further down the path. The question then is: how do you know what is in your best interest? The answer: by considering not just your fleeting preferences, but also how those wishes fit with the overall picture (i.e. your future hopes and dreams). There must be alignment between the two.

So who better to consult on this than your future self?

'Self' is a powerful force in human behaviour. Nearly every choice we make in life flows from our sense of who we are and what we believe is possible. It shapes the actions we are prepared to take and the magnitude of purpose we willingly pursue.

Hence, the more ardently a person can identify with their future self, the more likely they are to make the right choices.

To trust in your future self to the extent of letting it dictate your standards, beliefs and values now. That is acting 'as if' your 'future self' already, regardless of your current circumstances, and not somewhere to get to. 'Acting as if' can have the effect of invoking hidden reserves within us, inspiring us to live up to that ideal.

There's only one snag. For many of us, there's an emotional disconnect between 'present self' and 'future self.' Neuroscience teaches us we actually use different parts of our brain to think about our present self and our future self. In fact, when thinking about our future self, we activate our brain in the same way as thinking about a stranger. Nurturing a deeper connection with our future self then is like trying to empathise with another person, or at least a different person to whom we are now.

'Empathy' is traditionally defined as our ability to overcome our own perspective in order to appreciate the worldview of someone else. As it pertains to this instance; it becomes about overcoming our present self's perspective to include that held by future self. We can achieve this through mentally projecting ourselves into the future. The more often we can practise this, the more likely we are to establish a hearty *emphatic* connection with our future self.

On a practical level, a strong sense of 'future self' not only makes short-term sacrifices seem worthwhile but also makes the future appear more real and attainable. As a triathlete, I know this well. I always say fitting in and doing the training is the hard part. Race day is the fun part. There's the industrious 'present me' in training, invested in setting up 'future-self me' to race at my best on race day.

Another example of this principle is how I remind clients not to drink coffee after 4 pm, or drink that second or third glass of wine at night. Because whilst immediately satisfying, chances are it will lead to a largely sleepless or restless night. Fast forwarding to the next day, no doubt they would then perform sub-par. It helps provide a quick reality check by getting them to check in with their 'best self' before giving in to the temptation.

The reality is you are gifting yourself the satisfaction of tomorrow's rewards today. When you assume the long-term benefits are already yours, your brain then perceives missing out as a loss. You can verify this for yourself. How willing are you to give up on becoming your 'future self,' for the sake of 'instant gratification' today?

To sum up:

By regularly imagining, visualising and dwelling on our future self in vivid detail, we can condition ourselves to become more committed to that ideal.

And the greater our commitment to that future; the more we will find motivation, energy, and willpower in the present.

KEY CHAPTER TAKEAWAYS:

Get clear on WHO you really are. Keep evolving that identity by intentionally committing each day to the type of person you ultimately aspire to become.

Willpower (IDENTITY) leaks include limiting beliefs, unclear values, vague personal standards, self-criticism, ungratefulness, and arrogance.

Visualisation is a skill. Keep imagining your 'future self' until you can see yourself in vivid, expansive detail. Soon you will find yourself swept upstream by the strength of your conviction in future YOU, better prepared to face any unknowns.

5. WILLPOWER IS PART WAY POWER

Trying to willpower your way through every day only sets yourself up for eventual collapse. Facing too many - or repeatedly strong, temptations - ultimately leads to decision-fatigue, no matter your personal energy or motivational levels.

Far better to approach life like a smart athlete, learning to pace ourselves, gently testing and expanding our limits, and having a toolbox of proven SKILLS at our disposal.

This is the fun part now. This is where I present ways of bypassing willpower almost entirely. Some might call it *effortless* willpower.

The thinking being that by avoiding temptations wherever you can; you free up willpower for when you most need it.

1) The Press Pause Principal (delaying it by 20 minutes)

Tell yourself, 'not right now, but maybe later.' A momentary delay diverts attention off the part of your brain that wants it now.

The trick here is that during the 20 minute interval, find something to do, like go for a walk or drink some water. This helps put space between yourself and the temptation.

I do this with food. I tell myself if I still feel hungry in twenty minutes, then I might succumb. After a meal, this is often the time it takes for you to feel full or satiated, anyway. It helps lessen the immediate craving. Twenty minutes later, the urge is often not as strong, and I can go without or opt for a healthier alternative instead.

2) The Reset Principal (aligning your head and heart)

An extension of 'The Press Pause Principal' is adding breathing exercises to shift your body into a more optimal state. Anytime you press the upset button, you allow stress to hijack your thinking capacities. The alternative is to choose the reset option, based on the pause and plan work of Suzanne Segerstrom, a Professor in Clinical Psychology.

When faced with an internal conflict, your brain needs to bring your body on board with your goals. This is because your ability to pause and plan peaks when you are both calm (mentally) and relaxed (physically).

Pause. Breathe. Choose.

First, focus on breathing more from your belly than from your chest; then concentrate on slowing down your rate of breath. Just four to six breaths per minute, inhaling through your nose, exhaling through your mouth - for two to three minutes - can help move your brain and body from a state of stress to a state supportive of self-control.

When the promise of a reward takes over your brain, it releases dopamine to focus your attention and motivate you into action. The sequence of pausing, breathing slowly, and noticing what you are experiencing shuts this response down. It's inconsistent with the way the reward system operates, creating a functional disconnection. Soon, there is a balance between sympathetic and parasympathetic (autonomic nervous system) activation, plus equanimity of mind.

This positions you to choose how you would like to respond. What's the effort or cost involved? Is it worth your prime goal?! Run through the chain of consequences several times over in your mind. Ask yourself: How does taking this simple action now affect me in 10 mins - 10 hours - 10 days - 10 months - 10 years' time?

This trains that part of your mind responsible for foreseeing the consequences of any action. Plus, sometimes we're stopped more by fear than by a lack of willpower. Most importantly, you thinking it through means you make better decisions via aligning it with your higher-order intentions. It trains your mind to be at choice, rather than react on impulse, autopilot, or from external influence.

So in the heat of the moment, when you're feeling tempted or drained, remember that you may only be several deep breaths away from regaining your resolve. It also presents you with a window of time in which to make a different decision.

3) The Just Did It Principle

This employs the 'press pause principle' in reverse. Don't think about it. Do it. See how you go. See how you feel about doing it after 5 minutes have passed.

It's a misconception to think we must be in the right motivational state before beginning a task or activity. Often, it follows once we begin. Hence this principle nullifies the pain we might feel in anticipation of having to complete necessary work.

Of course, you can put any time limit on it you wish. Whatever constraint is sufficient in kick-starting you into doing something - that otherwise you might keep putting off - and that helps you build up momentum. The idea being that once you begin, you find yourself inspired or empowered to carry on. It works because getting started can not only change our perception of a task, but also that of our self.

An extension of this principle is to focus for longer and longer periods of time before giving into a distraction. Think of it as training your attention span not to give in to something more immediately gratifying. The reward being – you just did it!

4) The Out Of Sight – Out Of Mind Principle

Repeatedly resisting temptations drains willpower; so better to stay out of trouble in the first place. Simply hide the temptation or create distance or time between you and the temptation. Repeatedly denying yourself may suddenly lead to a downward spiral, as once you initially relapse, easy to tell yourself 'I might as well carry on now.' An obvious and well-known principle but would be amiss to omit it.

5) The Declutter Your Life Principle

This principle is the equivalent of temptation-proofing your environment: "When a flower doesn't bloom, you fix the environment in which it grows, not the flower."

Our brains process way more information today than back in the 1970s / 80s. The typical person ends up making about 2,000 decisions every waking hour. Even the most energetic of people don't have endless mental energy. Small, trivial choices, interruptions and mindless distractions all add up in terms of overall decision-fatigue.

It's why dieters can keep to a strict diet all day, only to relapse in the evening. It's also why we struggle to avoid engaging in "bad behaviours" when tempted by them over a long period. We waste willpower on non-essentials!

Thus, a big part of decluttering your life is organising and simplifying your days; thereby reducing the number of decisions you have to make and the options available to you. You will have less overall stress as a result, which will enable you to make wiser judgements. Less clutter also creates space for clarity and creativity to emerge.

Mainly though, it's about keeping your cognitive load low. Your working memory will increase as your cognitive load decreases, which will help you be less susceptible to sudden urges.

Try journaling and observing yourself for three days. Or if you can, seven days, as quite often weekends are different from weekdays.

Explore closely late afternoons and evenings, as that's when you're more vulnerable to slipping up.

How might you eliminate willpower-draining triggers or activities?

Where can you automate decisions or remove or hide temptations?

Where can you routinize aspects of your life you consider mundane?

Any behaviour that can be reduced to a routine or habit is one less behaviour that we must spend time and energy consciously thinking about and deciding upon.

Examples include pre-set meals for the entire week; wear the same clothes or the same colours three days at a time; workout to a pre-set programme; or toss a coin as to which film to watch on live streaming instead of studying the reviews beforehand etc.

6) The Reduce / Increase Friction Principle

This principle is about making it easy to take the right actions and hard to take the wrong ones.

Think: how can you make the right choice the 'default' option, even when you're hungry, tired, stressed, or rushed?

Reduce Friction:
- Plan your workouts. Lay your clothes out the night before an early morning gym trip.

- Take up a gym membership in winter months, to guard against inclement weather.

- Stock your kitchen up with healthy snacks. Have fresh fruit on display. Hide crisps and biscuits away. Prepare meals at the weekend for weekdays. Avoid all-you-can-eat buffets.

- Stay hydrated. Store filtered water in a glass bottle. Keep it visible throughout the day.

- Add a new behaviour on to an existing behaviour. e.g. If you finish your working day at 6 pm with a green tea or carbohydrate drink, then plan your run straight after that.

A Quick Note on Habits

The right habits are equivalent to delegating choices to autopilot. Once established, they require little maintenance. Hence, it's almost too obvious not to include them under 'reducing friction.' Developing habits is a self-regulating process itself, and is therefore to be encouraged, to an extent. By that, I don't believe anyone should go to the extreme of setting up habits to account for 100 percent of their behaviours in life and work.

Just because the human brain is designed so people can do things without having to think, doesn't imply routine should rule your life. The frontal lobes are the largest lobes in the human brain for good reason. Apart from separating us from other creatures on this earth, they enable us to carry out higher-level executive functions such as predicting, planning, organising, and self-monitoring etc. Yes, in short, thinking! Why waste such a valuable resource?

Rant aside; using willpower to develop adaptive habits is a good use of willpower, as long as you don't get carried away. Chances are you won't, anyway; as it's well known that many people struggle to accumulate good habits. Much has been written on the subject already. Here, I'll just reiterate the key contributory factors to successful habit-building:

Add one habit at a time. Piggyback a new habit onto an existing habit if you can. Stay focused on how many total days you've completed your habit. If you do lapse, identify where it fell apart for you, and then go again. Gift yourself small, simple and healthy rewards along the way. Immediate reinforcement improves intrinsic motivation and increases the likelihood you will sustain the habit.

Your choice of reward must be valued by you personally. The more immediate the better, since we value instant over delayed rewards. Allow yourself to savour the positive feelings it creates. Suitable choices include: relaxing in the sun - a coffee break - a hot bubble bath – your favourite music – the latest movie - a hobby - a chapter of a book - a podcast - a game with a friend - journaling or reflection time - or a walk in nature.

Increase Friction
- Keep less healthy food in hard to reach places (out of sight).

- No more than 1 or 2 wine bottles in your house (at any one time).

- Delete your credit cards from websites (so you have to constantly re-enter your information each time you shop).

- Clean your teeth after your evening meal (to stop yourself snacking at night).

- Place a strict 2 hour limit on TV + social media time each day.

Please note: Situational strategies work especially well for physical temptations (e.g., junk food) that can be avoided, hidden, or made inconvenient.

7) The If-Then Principle

This is one of my favourite principles and a tool of mine added to the toolbox at Positivepsychology.com in 2017.

The 'If-then' principle works by anticipating obstacles in advance. This allows you to prepare and plan for them beforehand, when presumably your willpower is higher. Accepting you will undoubtedly face temptations can help weaken the strength of a temptation when it does arise. By foreseeing when, where and how temptation might strike, you can plan specific actions to overcome them ahead of time. Perhaps even look for ways to avoid them altogether.

Look for patterns. What triggers temptation for you: Certain times, places, events, people? Plan ahead. Visualize the process. What steps are needed to reach your goal? Sometimes just picturing each step in the process can make it appear easier and reduce anxiety. Then here's the formula: "If X happens, then Y."

Where: X can be a time, place, event. And Y is the specific action you will take if X occurs.

Example One: If I sleep badly two consecutive nights, then I will have a quiet evening in (with laptop off by 8 pm) and be in bed by 10 pm.

Example Two: If I end up working late today, then I'll wake up 30 minutes earlier tomorrow to go for a run before having breakfast (to make up for missing my gym workout).

Rather than navigate each scenario in your head at the time, you simply plan ahead for various contingencies and pre-decide or commit to a course of action in advance.

The 'If-Then Principle' works well for any intention, even big ones. Anytime you dream up a positive vision of the future, look to offset it by thinking through any potential challenges that may arise. Some might call it 'realistic optimism': High expectations on the one hand, counter-balanced by the wisdom you will likely face difficulties in achieving it.

8) The Exaggeration Principle

Let's say you begin writing, and within a few minutes, you get an urge. You want to check your phone, just in case someone has messaged you or there's breaking news. Pause for a moment. Make what this is costing you sound explicit. Tell yourself: "I'm not just wasting a few seconds. I'm taking chunks out of my working day, which adds up over a week. Soon, I'm likely to fall short of my main goals. If that happens, I not only disappoint myself but I let other people around me down, who stand by and believe in me."

You get the gist. You turn something seemingly trivial into something titanic. Small actions can have cascading consequences. By exaggerating the consequences in your mind, you hopefully dial down the appeal of the current distraction.

Another example of this principle is using the power of 'contrast.' e.g. would you rather… 'make time for wellness, or make time for illness?' or 'get enough sleep, or make frequent mistakes?' or 'choose healthy eating habits, or struggle with your weight?' Have fun with this one making up some of your own.

9) The Temptation Bundling Principle

Temptation-bundling can happen in different forms. One example is where you pair pleasure with a delayed reward. For instance, this could be exercising whilst also listening to an audiobook. This way you get to listen to an audiobook that you desperately want to find the time to listen to. It also combats procrastinating on the exercise side, since the benefits of exercise are not always immediately obvious.

I often bribe myself by using this technique. Like allowing myself to watch a 90 minute football game ONLY if I'm spinning away on a bike at the same time. One activity I want to do; the other, I know I should do to maintain my level of fitness, but is time-consuming. Hence, doing both would not be an option. Instead, it's an appropriate compromise. Or if cycling with friends, we only get to stop for coffee and cake, if we first put in a hard effort on the bike. We have to earn it.

Another example of this principle is pairing an undesirable or non-urgent task with an attractive one. Maybe filing or organising paperwork whilst listening to your favourite music. It's a way to reward yourself for doing something you need to do, but would rather not do. Think how you might transform an energy-draining task into an energy-giving activity or before using up precious willpower, see if you can make your actions more appealing to do.

10) The Alter Ego Principle

This one was based on 'The Alter Ego Effect,' published by Todd Herman in 2019. A principle I was aware of, being a competitive athlete, but didn't have a name for. Just like Superman, Wonder Woman and Spiderman have two versions of themselves; we each have a hidden heroic or best Self. A source of latent power in various forms: creativity, resourcefulness, mental toughness or curiosity, etc.

It will differ from person to person. The principle though is to build your alter-ego into a character, congruent with your purpose and values. For me, my nickname is 'IronNoel,' since I've completed an Ironman. It's then traditional in triathlon to be called 'Iron-YOURNAME.'

I'm also a lifelong supporter of West Ham who are nicknamed the 'Irons.' This means that when I require it, such as struggling in training or racing, I quickly visualise and summon upon 'IronNoel' - my Alter Ego. It's that strong version of me who has been there before and knows how to dig deep, that believes 'pain is temporary; victory is forever!' Please don't laugh. It works 95% of the time. With this in mind, what will your Alter Ego be?!

11) The Single Focus Principle

This principle is about concentrating 100% on the task at hand. Sometimes even the most committed of us don't feel like exercising. It could be the weather, our to-do list that day, a buildup from previous training sessions, a lack of quality sleep, etc. Whatever the case, sometimes you have to dig a little deeper than other days. The Single Focus Principle helps by blotting everything else out of my mind, knowing it can all wait until I've finished what I'm doing now. That way, I'm fully present in the moment, going all-in. It helps completely clear the mind, allowing it to focus purely on the task-at-hand.

It's also an example of what's known as 'the Stockdale paradox' (based on former Vietnam POW, James Stockdale). I'm able to accept my current 'uncomfortable' reality because of the faith I have in the long-term rewards of exercising regularly. It helps provide a frame for adopting a dual present-and-future focus that effectively channels willpower.

12) The Social Accountability Principle

The final principle in this chapter is about going public and bringing on board other people to keep you on track.

You see people on social networks announcing their intentions or goals in public, and then relying on the support and encouragement of others to see them through to completion.

There's a reason too Strava is popular for sharing exercise training sessions. The fact other people see your work-out stats can spur you on to do the session, instead of skipping it. Also, it spurs you on to push yourself harder or longer than you might have done, if no-one else got to see. Plus, when you see what other people - just like you - are doing, it can inspire you to push yourself equally hard. It helps bring out the competitor in you.

So there you go - twelve principles to help you bypass willpower. Admittedly, there are some overlaps. However, the main intention was to stimulate your thinking and hopefully for you to conjure up some principles of your own.

KEY CHAPTER TAKEAWAYS:

Facing too many - or repeatedly strong - temptations leads to decision-fatigue.

With the right SKILLS, you can bypass the need for willpower in the moment.

The number of ways you can modify your mindset and personal situation are limited only by your imagination. If you feel stuck, reach out to a coach or mentor to assist you.

6. WILLPOWER IS PART WHY POWER

The premise behind 'Why Power' is that with the right motivation, less willpower is required. In addition, higher levels of motivation can compensate for 'depleted' willpower reserves. This can be achieved through any combination of the following:

INTENSIFY YOUR VISION

When you intensify your vision - by making it both concrete and captivating - you are more likely to remain loyal to it, long after the initial inspiration has vanished.

Remember in chapter one, we said your brain is biased in prioritising immediate guaranteed rewards over delayed rewards. This present bias means we would rather settle for a smaller immediate reward than wait for a larger future reward. This happens because your reward system creates the promise of a reward so strong (think food temptations!), that it's easy to stop paying attention to the regret of the consequences.

However, what researchers have also observed is that when people waited for a reward, there was increased activity in the region of the brain that helped them think about the future (the anterior prefrontal cortex). More patient individuals, it seems, devote more energy to imagining receiving their reward later. This suggests anticipation matters. The more compelling and concrete that future reward, the more likely we are to wait for it. In contrast, fuzzy imaging only serves to distort our thinking about distant rewards, and the effort required in obtaining them.

The power in future visioning then is being able to intensify our future desire, over and above the appeal of our present desire - e.g. a fit body by Summer or tasty, comfort food now in Winter? So, before yielding to any temptation, try dwelling on your desired future instead for a few minutes. See if it can help you overcome the immediate urge, by refocusing you. Jim Rohn, the American philosopher, summed the dilemma up succinctly when he said you have two choices: The price of discipline or the pain of regret.

Michelle Segar, an American behavioural sustainability scientist, framed it as 'chore versus gift.' I.e. reframe your chosen behaviour as a beneficial opportunity, rather than an obligation or burden. Ask yourself, 'why am I going to eat well, be physically active and get good night of sleep today (i.e. the chore)? Answer, because I know it helps me look and feel GREAT (i.e. the gift).

Ideally too your desire to achieve this vision would be intrinsically driven i.e. something you want to do for its own sake, because it means something personally to you. Indeed, when your vision is aligned with your Identity and congruent with your values, exerting willpower can seem almost 'effortless'. Whereas pursuing outcomes, that are not as well-internalized, requires effort. So whilst doing what you value can take effort, it's even harder to push yourself to do what you do not fully stand behind. See Quirin et al. (March 2021) in Further Reading.

To sum up, a captivating vision (e.g. enchanting; intrinsically driven; aligned with your identity; congruent with your values) not only leads to less willpower depletion, but can also elevate your overall vitality.

I think this is why many people find it beneficial to make time daily (say 10-15 min) for deep reflection on their primary goals, thus accentuating their desirability. Plus, why fast forwarding and contemplating your future self is equally valuable.

BECOME PURPOSE-DRIVEN

"Enthusiasm is common. Endurance is rare." – Angela Duckworth.

A sense of purpose helps give your intentions an emotional edge. Abstract goals don't grab us for long. The key lies in being able to find the right motive. Not something we 'should' change, but that we genuinely 'want' to. Perhaps something that reinforces our future self (our aspiration for who we wish to become), whilst stimulating learning, challenge and personal growth.

Here's why that is important. Not only can dedication buffer against everyday struggles; those same aggravations can provoke a stronger, more authentic, purpose in our lives. We can grow from the experience, sometimes even finding a new direction to follow. I watched a super video from Victor Strecher, a professor at the University of Michigan's School of Public Health, explaining this. He illustrated how the ventral medial PFC area of the brain is active when self-affirming core purposeful values and how this then guides decision-making. Such neural firing also down-regulates activity in the amygdala, which would explain how purpose might buffer against stress.

A strong enough conviction in a worthwhile cause can also help fill endless cravings and lessen distractions. Because the more we give of ourselves, the less we seem to crave, especially if we can get behind an endeavour beyond or bigger than us. Committing to the 'greater common good' expands our sense of compassion with other people and the world as a whole. It helps make purpose even more potent, fostering energy and resilience, while deterring lethargy and self-absorption.

Finally, committing to a purpose is the equivalent of choosing ahead of time. Instantly gratifying; it creates good feelings in advance. So when you next feel low on willpower, reflect and remind yourself WHY your intentions matter so much.

THE POWER OF PRE-COMMITMENT

"People with low willpower use it to get themselves out of crises. People with high willpower use it NOT to get themselves into crises." – Roy Baumeister.

A pre-commitment refers to deciding your priorities in advance. When you reduce your number of choices, you reduce your willpower demands. Plus, when you make a decision ahead of time, you don't waste energy by repeatedly deliberating it. Further, it often proves easier to decide in advance what you will do versus fending off temptation in the heat of the moment.

An often hidden yet obvious secret to willpower is sound mental discipline. Simply put, many of us have too much going on. An overloaded mind is also a highly distractible mind. In contrast, a focused, committed mind is better positioned to exert willpower. So dedicate yourself to one project at a time and see it through to completion. Willpower is misdirected if it's in constant use or if it's applied to something you are not 100% committed to.

People with the highest self-control are the ones who call upon willpower, only when warranted, in pursuit of their biggest, boldest goals.

Pre-commitments then are a means of aligning with your highest self in order to establish your most worthy goals. Your best 'future self' demands you pursue only priority projects. Pre-commitments represent a way of asking your 'future self' to honour them too. So make the decision: YES or NO. Then go all in. Because once your present self has committed, you lock yourself on a virtuous path. And with a strong enough commitment, there's both a will and a way.

There's an additional bonus too. The visionary ability to see events before they happen - to 'see everything twice' - puts you ahead of the game. You gain confidence from feeling prepared and are also less likely to act on impulse.

VALUING DIFFICULTY

'Satisfaction lies in the effort, not in the attainment; full effort is full victory.' - Mahatma Gandhi

There are some people with high levels of willpower who equate 'difficult' with worthwhile. These individuals are motivated to pursue challenges precisely because they require considerable effort. They see discomfort not only as part of the exchange, but also as potentially rewarding, relative to something that can be achieved with little effort. The mere act of taking on a slightly daunting challenge can lead to a surge in personal energy in these daring people. What then might be a struggle for one person can be viewed as a worthwhile challenge by another (e.g., running a marathon or racing in a triathlon) and enjoyable to relive again afterwards.

Finding value in effort is how we can find hidden reserves of strength toward the end of a race. The effort itself becomes rewarding, with neuroimaging supporting this. It has been shown that the ventral striatum (i.e., a brain region involved in processing rewarding outcomes) is more strongly activated when we achieve something through higher effort than lower effort. Of course, being able to 'do hard' is advantageous when pursuing any personally valued but difficult goal. Plus, people who derive enjoyment from effort report higher life satisfaction and meaning as well.

In contrast, if we have less faith in willpower and believe that it's foolish to try too hard, then we are liable to downsize the goals we set for ourselves. The thing is, 'easy' goals tend to get us the same old results. Plus, as individuals, we don't change or grow much in the process. On top of that, it can affect our level of personal well-being in that we start to feel less empowered to go after what we really want in life. If a goal requires little effort, we can quickly lose the motivation to pursue it. I quote Dr. Andrew Huberman: 'if everyone is rewarded to the same level (every participant gets a trophy), the value of the prize is diminished, and the value of effort to achieve that thing also diminishes.'

This is why it's important to keep the faculty of effort alive in you. To tap into willpower most days by holding yourself accountable to do what's most important, although not necessarily easy. Maybe even to try something new or to override a habitual way of doing something. Repeated small acts of willpower in one domain, even when seemingly inconsequential, can contribute to available willpower in other areas: emotional control, spending, social media usage, foods and drinks, and household chores. It's partly why I maintain a competitive level of fitness and a rigorous training schedule today. I find it helps keep me motivated and focused in life in general, not to mention less stressed and in better health.

Regular physical exercise is essentially little more than repeated acts of willpower. It coaxes our ability to tolerate various degrees of distress. It's important to remember too that you've always got a little bit more than you think you have. Most limits are self-imposed by our mind, which seeks to protect our brain and body. Apparently, US Navy SEALs hold fast to a 40% rule: 'When you think you're at your limit of exhaustion, you actually have 60% of your energy reserves left'. Personally, I find it helpful to adapt this rule by breaking any run or bike course down into sections. I get so far, then recollect myself, then go again. It's easier on the mind than thinking about the course as a whole, and I get more out of myself.

Just like exercise fatigues you, using willpower may quickly tire it. If your willpower is 'out of shape,' then expect to work a little harder just to get your self-control back up to optimal levels again. Then it should become easier. Even just knowing it should get easier with time may help you muster up some willpower today. What defines 'hard' is often more a mental battle than it is physical. For example, most people quit too soon with exercise. If you stick with it, exercising does get easier. You have to give the psychological and physical benefits a chance to kick in until it becomes your new normal. Also, at first, don't attempt your most difficult willpower challenge. Start with the smallest change consistent with moving towards your main goal. Train your willpower there and look to build your strength back up.

Another factor to consider is this: If we believe it will get easier, we are more likely to persist. This is in some ways self-fulfilling, in that by persisting, we grow in commitment and confidence, and it does start to feel easier.

All things considered, then, it's both possible and advantageous to learn to develop a level of tolerance for distress. Adopting such a mindset is invaluable in that most things in life are oftentimes harder than they look, or not as fun as they first appear. By stretching ourselves again and again; we can bring out the best in ourselves. Besides actively leaning into challenges and getting comfortable with being somewhat uncomfortable, this is generally what it takes to go after the bigger goals in life anyhow. Plus, keep in mind that the fear of failing is usually more intense than any pain felt following an actual failure. As Goethe remarked, 'Whatever you can do or dream you can, begin it; boldness has genius, power, and magic in it.' So try embracing a little difficulty in your life. You might just end up surprising yourself!

That said, whilst embracing challenges can be a good thing, take care not to overdo it. Attempting too much can lead to frustration, burnout, and even mental health issues. There's a balance to be found.

FINDING FLOW

Overcoming challenges requires creativity. It's intriguing then that challenge and creativity are also the two key triggers for inducing the 'flow' state. Because if ever willpower could be described as effortless, it's when we experience flow.

Flow is the positive mental state that occurs when we are so completely immersed in an activity that we lose our sense of 'self' and awareness of 'time'. The equivalent of motivation squared. Also known as being 'in the zone,' flow is triggered when your current skill level is appropriately challenged (i.e., usually in the region of 1-4% incremental improvement).

Essentially, in this state, we trade higher cognitive functions for heightened attention and awareness. This puts any decisions on autopilot, with minimal second-guessing; meaning the need for willpower is negligible.

Therein is the attraction of flow: It's a highly rewarding and desirable state to find yourself in, at little cost to you personally. The trouble is it's not that easy to find flow amongst the hustle and bustle of modern life; nor should you expect to be able to stay in the flow state for long. Like anything in life, it occurs in cycles. It's also a bit like aspiring to be happy 24/7 – it's just not realistic for multiple reasons.

DEVELOPING A WINNING (CAN DO) ATTITUDE
Positive attitudes may buffer the effects of mild willpower depletion, and help both steel and fortify your resolve in the face of obstacles.

Just some of the recognised traits of a winning attitude to consider are:
- Ambitious (driven by a desire to achieve more than others)
- Laser-like Clarity (lucid predictions of intended outcomes)
- Determined (self-responsible for actions)
- Realistic Optimism (expecting challenges; recovering quickly from adversity)
- Unwavering Belief (upbeat in the face of adversity; setbacks are springboards)
- Committed (clear and confident that the prize is worth both the cost and sacrifice)
- Intrinsic Generosity (a giver rather than a taker)
- Flexible Thinking (outperforms black-or-white thinking)
- Focused (not allowing external influences to impact existing motivation).

How do you score? Each winner will have a different combination of these characteristics that assist in driving and steering them onward to success.

Note that a winning attitude is not always something that can be learned from books. It generally has to be earned through life experience.

KEY CHAPTER TAKEAWAYS:

The right MOTIVATION can be a powerful ally in overcoming depleted willpower. There's power in being pulled by a compelling vision or mighty purpose.

Pre-commitment refers to deciding your priorities in advance, so as not to be led into temptation.

It's important to keep the faculty of exerting effort alive in you at healthy levels. A positive attitude can buffer mild willpower depletion.

7. 10X YOUR WILLPOWER WITH WE POWER

"What differentiates us as a social species is the need to be seen and known and loved, and the need to see and know and love others." – Brené Brown.

We-power encompasses not only good physical and psychological health but also meaningful relationships with other people (realized through common values and feeling like a substantial part of a broader social environment). All of which has relevance with regards to strengthening our individual willpower.

WILLPOWER IS BIGGER THAN SELF

We are all wired to be social, mixing within various societal cultures. As such, SELF is never created in isolation. Our external environment shapes our personal identity on a daily basis, contributing to a sense of belonging to something bigger than us. What's more, the people and networks we associate with are constantly rewiring our brains and our minds - for better or worse.

WILLPOWER IS CONTAGIOUS (FRIEND POWER)

Studies have shown that participants who share positive psychology activities with significant others experience a motivational lift. Not only do their significant others benefit but participants do too - in terms of amplified positive effects - relative to carrying out the exercises alone. Similarly, sometimes it's easier to walk or run with others than it is to drag yourself out alone. We know too that rowers or cyclists are likely to push themselves more and workout harder when in a group.

We also know that the brain has mirror neurons that automatically track what other people are thinking, feeling, and doing. These mirror neurons automatically help us better understand the emotions and intentions of other people. This might explain why we become like the people we spend the most time with. Perhaps even 'the average of your five closest friends,' according to motivational speaker Jim Rohn.

It's no secret, then, that the fastest way to change yourself is to hang out with people you aspire to be like. Someone who has accomplished what you want to do. Willpower comes from role models, peers, and friends who both care about you and incite you to tap into their inner strength. Even just thinking about someone with high self-control, and doing so frequently, can increase your own. Individual willpower is thus powerfully shaped by social influence - the people who surround us.

"The influence of a vital person vitalizes" - Joseph Campbell.

THE POWER OF SOCIAL SUPPORT

Digging deeper, social support is a source of nourishment in itself, impacting well-being and life satisfaction as much as the big three of sleep, diet, and exercise. Feeling well-connected boosts our motivation, meaning, and willpower. In turn, willpower improves our social relationships reinforcing the bidirectional effect. Positive social relationships also prompt the body to produce neurochemicals that reduce stress and anxiety and help lower cortisol levels and inflammation. Social connection also strengthens our immune system.

Not least of all, social activity adds enjoyment to life. Relationships help you open up, become wiser and more attuned, as well as boost your resilience, happiness and health. In addition, pursuing meaningful personal goals is rewarding in itself. Connecting with others in that pursuit can only add to the rewards. Finally, being supportive of others brings out the best in us and uplifts everyone by breeding a collective, positive spirit of unleashing potential.

Going it alone can prove costly
Conversely, a lack of strong social connections can negatively impact your health, similar in risk to that of smoking. Feeling lonely or socially isolated can make you more prone to depression, impulsivity, and addiction. No surprise then that social exclusion

exerts a double whammy effect: Your willpower is diminished. Your cravings feel stronger than ever. Not a good place to be! What's fascinating too is that when you feel socially excluded, you activate the same regions in your brain that respond to physical pain — the insula and the anterior cingulate cortex. For many, it's both psychologically and physically harmful to feel separated or excluded from significant others.

NURTURING A SUPPORTIVE ENVIRONMENT AROUND YOU

It follows that the smartest way to navigate life is by being part of a supportive collective that has each other's backs. Irritations and challenges are largely an inevitable part of life. Hence, surrounding yourself with friends or upbeat people, who encourage and better you, can be a potent tool for maintaining personal standards and keeping stress at bay.

"There's just one way to radically change your behaviour: radically change your environment." — B.J. Fogg.

So first, be grateful for all the people currently inside your inner circle of support and influence. Next, ask yourself: Do they all help inspire you? Or do some dilute or drain you? Where might you benefit from bolstering your support, and in what area? For instance, you could sign up with any number of existing clubs, groups, and local or online communities.

Alternatively, you could find other people with the same goal(s) and start a supportive group yourself. We can gain strength, as well as know-how, by helping others make the changes we often want for ourselves!

Think about how you might prove useful to others and ideally to many. See it as adding to their social support network before wanting or needing anything in return. It's a step up from indulgent self-help and self-absorption or being the brightest light shining. Instead, it becomes a collective pursuit and the coming together of a bunch of bright lights. Knowing who's there to inspire, guide, help, or replenish you, increases that all-in-it-together spirit. It equips you to face up better to challenges and adversity. Surrounded by people who understand, value, elevate, and support us; we feel anything is possible.

This is powerful in that bold or big goals aren't often achieved all at once, or without experiencing discouraging setbacks along the way. Willpower is so much easier when you don't go it alone.

EVOKING EXCELLENCE IN OTHERS:

To sum up, we often blame ourselves for having low willpower, but modern living is a breeding ground for energy depletion.

Our choices are influenced by our surroundings far more than we might think or believe. Social norms greatly influence individual levels of self-control. Ironically, we witness this effect strongest in reverse. The statistics show that being overweight or obese spreads through families, friends, and social connections like a virus.

The good news is that believing we can meaningfully contribute to other people and to the world around us improves our sense of well-being. As does feeling we can access support for ourselves in return. Both sides of the equation (e.g., giving and receiving) are important in the strengthening of social bonds.

In improving the communities in which we live, strong bonds also enhance societal well-being. High levels of individual willpower add up across an entire community with the capability to advance the greater good. Just like a rising tide lifts all boats, willpower is a social strength that can uplift us all. Perhaps that's why leading social psychologist Roy Baumeister deemed it the 'greatest human strength?

Willpower can pull us out of the 'daily grind' and put our minds on better things.

With the socially-minded values of previous generations on the wane, I trust I am not alone in thinking that the prosocial concept of willpower - as a source of social strength - is of paramount significance today!

KEY CHAPTER TAKEAWAYS:

Self-control is heavily influenced by social control.

Your SURROUNDINGS, and the level of social support you both generate and receive, can increase your willpower success.

In turn, willpower is a valuable social strength, leading to prosocial behaviours.

8 UNLEASHING RESERVES OF WILLPOWER

'To be yourself in a world that is constantly trying to make you something else is the greatest accomplishment.' - Ralph Waldo Emerson.

So far, each chapter has examined the numerous ways that neurobiology, biology, identity, skills, motivation, and your surroundings shape willpower. It's the dynamic interplay between all these parts that gives rise to the energy or strength we call willpower. As such, I hope you now see that willpower is not something simply bestowed on you. It includes additional domains you can manage and protect.

Willpower = WellPower + WhoPower + WayPower + WhyPower + WePower

In this chapter, I'll now attempt to sum up the lessons learned throughout this guidebook with some additional practical observations. With simplicity as ever in mind, let's say there are three key pillars for optimising willpower: self-care, self-awareness, and self-determination.

1) SELF-CARE

You can't expect to have reserves of willpower if you're depleted mentally, emotionally, or physically. Hence, it starts with assembling good self-care habits (i.e., WELL power) and the right social support (i.e., SOCIAL power) in a manner that works well for you and for those around you. The cumulative benefits pave the way for a clearer and calmer state of mind, coupled with improved mood and brain function. Signs of positivity, high energy levels, feelings of empowerment, and strong interpersonal relationships are all reminders that you are on track and that you have in place the necessary foundational pillars for willpower.

2) SELF-AWARENESS

Today our minds can be stimulated or distracted 24/7, meaning you never need stop and check in with yourself, if you don't want to. It's easy for our inner voice to get drowned out by all the external noise and constant stimulation. Whilst this might plaster over the ordinariness of mundane living, it could also be blocking us from uncovering our most authentic selves and where that might lead us in life.

Reclaiming control of your mental and emotional faculties is then crucial in determining your ability to choose. After all, is free will not about ownership of your own mind? It's also your means of living in integrity with your WHO and your WHY. Higher levels of self-awareness help reinforce your identity (i.e., you at your core). This in turn inherently reinforces your confidence levels, well-being, and strength of social relationships, etc.

Every day your immediate surroundings are shaping your decisions and actions, often accidentally, at any given moment. As a result, traditional cognitive willpower strategies can easily be reversed by your environment. Yet they put the burden on you, the individual. One way to counter this is to prune away the excess (e.g., physical stuff, distractions, reactive people, endless entertainment, too many commitments, etc.). In a world of limitless options, it pays to be picky when the tendency is to gravitate towards 'more.' It's 'less,' though, that helps us hone in better on our vision, radiate our authenticity, and live into our highest potential.

Maybe because it's difficult to connect with and access your true self, when it's buried deep beneath busyness, stresses, and distractions. Besides consuming valuable time and energy, it may also prevent boredom from progressing to a state where we give ourselves time and space for contemplation. Boredom and mind-wandering provide a fertile foundation for creativity, which is why many good ideas come to us in the shower or while traveling from A to B. Just look at the recent pandemic lockdowns. There was a common urge to fill the emptiness. New passions or hobbies were discovered, and new careers or directions in life were chosen.

Additionally, a deeper self-bond is integral to connecting better with other humans and the world at large. As opposed to the more recognised, crystallized intelligence, it leads to fluid intelligence. Namely, a heightened awareness of what's going on, both inside and around you. Plus the ability to think on your feet when surrounded by uncertainty, complexity, or conflict, all assisted by a constant marvel at and curiosity about life in general. Most significantly, it puts you back in control, taking responsibility for choosing and staying on the right track. All in all, self-awareness enhances your ability to live intentionally, ensuring your choices are consistent and congruent with your best interests.

3) SELF DETERMINATION

 # Step One: Know what you (really) want.
Problems in life are not due to low self-esteem. We only undermine ourselves by spotting deficits and then attempting to fix whatever we feel is lacking. Why? Because the issue with 'thinking well of yourself' is that it involves constant recalibration. We can find ourselves subject to the whims of external forces or in need of more and more fixes, like a boat that's sinking. We liberate ourselves by shifting our focus. Knowing 'what we really want' is the main motivator in life.

It then becomes less about you, and more about whatever you are directing your energies towards. It kicks in and capitalises on parts of your neurobiology that make it harder for you to stop. Soon you start to feel more responsive in the face of life events, expertly adjusting to them in pursuit of your goals. This fuels a willingness to persist, as you step-by-step build faith in yourself and strengthen your convictions in whatever you are choosing to pursue.

> "Willpower is more than your ability to say NO.
> It's the strength of your determination behind a bigger YES."

Exerting willpower for autonomous reasons (i.e., yours) requires less effort than acting on what you think you should do. Accordingly, whittle your wants down to what you want and clarify your why. Then answer the call - to goals that excite but test you, that give more than they take. To goals that have meaning and purpose for you and that align with your values. By committing yourself 100%, you eliminate room for negotiation (a known willpower wrecker).

So step one: Gain clarity on your desired ultimate outcome.

Step Two: Expect obstacles.

Of course, resistance will surface, testing your clarity of vision, strength of motivation, level of commitment, and social support. This is to be expected.

> 'Say YES to temporary discomfort,
> so you can say NO to a lifetime of regrets.'

The road to success is rarely straight. Everybody experiences resistance, in all walks of life. Everybody has up and down days. The difference is aspiring to become bigger than our problems, accepting certain limitations with self-compassion, and striving to be better. Once you get this, it becomes easier to start walking your path in life, just taking your next best step as it arises. As Mother Teresa once wisely said, 'Be faithful in small things, because it is in them that your strength lies.'

Step two then is to see encountering challenges as part of the path. Not signals to stop. Appreciate each hurdle for being there, sculpting you, and nudging you into finding out who you really are. Keep reaching for worthwhile goals that stretch you, knowing it's how we all evolve and grow into increasingly extraordinary human beings.

Step Three: Conserve willpower.

If willpower is exhausted through constant or hard usage, it is best to reserve willpower for your most important challenges only.

Set your life up in such a way that you are in a position of being able to apply willpower sparingly. Willpower is wasted on stuff that doesn't really matter.

So if something isn't important to you, eliminate it. Simplify and streamline your life on an ongoing basis. It's about recognising who you are and what you stand for in the context of your own life. No social comparisons then necessary. By intentionally aligning your actions with your future aspirations, you can determine where your attention and energy are best directed. It may mean making some tough calls!

I quote philosopher Alessandra Buccella: 'Only a small subset of our everyday actions is important enough to worry about.' This meme lies at the heart of essentialism. The majority of us are too busy, just trying to keep up, to pinpoint what truly matters to us in life. Others frown upon the idea of 'simplifying' or 'decluttering', since it would seem to contradict the popular ideal of 'having it all.' Nonetheless, it can prove incredibly liberating for those who are willing.

It can also prove less costly. Overwhelm and apathy are the prices we pay for not clearly setting out our priorities in life. Also, when we are feeling overloaded or jaded, we are more likely to find distractions that redirect our minds toward 'easier' tasks that our 'old self' is familiar with or proficient at. It's simply less demanding. But in doing so, we deprive ourselves of the chance to grasp what needs to be learned in order to move us one step closer towards our desired future.

To sum up, step three is to choose your willpower battles wisely so as to free up vital mental space for accurate thinking and decision-making. This leads us into step four.

Step Four: Apply willpower judiciously.

The real secret behind willpower is perhaps not a secret at all.

Those with the most self-control only exert willpower when they have to and where it is most needed.

Such cases can be grouped into three convenient categories:

a) For staying 'on task' when pursuing specific, short-term goals that you feel compelled to do rather than want to do.

b) For upholding your core values and personal standards. There must be something worthwhile in it. Pain without gain wastes willpower.

c) For achieving long-term goals, which are more susceptible to ongoing opposition (e.g., temptation, procrastination, diminished motivation) and thus require extra dedication and resources.

Some people will feel their willpower is strong, justified by how many urges, impulses, and temptations they are able to resist each day. The counterargument here is that willpower is being overused. You should not put yourself in that position in the first place. Your energy, passion, and strengths are better directed elsewhere.

There's a super research paper on this theme – please see Irving (2022) in Further Reading. Better self-regulation (i.e., self-management; managing your 'stress' load, etc.) helps make self-control unnecessary or possible (i.e., greater reserves are available when willpower is called for).

Step Five: See willpower as a superpower.

Change is not a one-time event, and the world is arguably moving faster now than ever before in history. Growth must therefore be chosen again and again. We can't afford to stay where we are for very long. Adopting this mindset can support us in thinking and operating in growth-oriented ways, which in turn optimises the constant rewiring of our brains (e.g., neuroplasticity). The earlier we adopt this mindset in life - constantly probing and expanding our limits - the better. Each choice then accrues compound interest, whilst signalling a commitment to all future choices, and the type of person we aspire to become.

Consequently, when we frame willpower as 'helping us to execute on our priorities even when they seem more difficult,' we are in effect endorsing a growth mindset. Viewing challenges as growth opportunities means we will try something AND persevere if we have to. In rising to each occasion, we gain strength. By purposefully embracing difficulties, and facing-up to any conflicting feelings that arise, we evolve as human beings. Through it, we revive or build inner strengths (e.g. patience, courage, confidence, clarity, resilience), which help us get things done, navigate challenges, and live a richer life. Seen in this light, willpower is a superpower. It enables us to go after what we want, coupled with the resolve to stay on the 'right' path, thereby minimising regret. It's a vital ingredient in 'mental toughness', in believing that the future will work out well for us.

Over and above that, arduous passages light the way to a more fully-integrated self, affording us greater freedom over the direction of our lives. Struggles, trials, tribulations, setbacks, etc. are all part of the ride and ultimately necessary components in revealing or sculpting who we become. A safety-orientated life, based around comfort, convenience, ease and quiet, is unlikely to reveal much about us. Except perhaps which character qualities we are lacking. We all have to 'battle' away somewhat in life, for our true or best selves to emerge.

As psychotherapist Stephen Cope has described it: 'personal fulfillment happens not in *retreat* from the world, but in *advance* — from profound engagement.' It's how inner strengths are forged, vision gets clarified, and ambition is inspired. We all have that choice, to be our real selves (i.e., inspired), or to retreat (i.e., be survival-led).

Yes, it is human nature to fear loss and protect ourselves from collecting life's battle scars. Instead, we must train our minds to embrace the gain – that is, of becoming who deep down we aspire to become. To one day, on our deathbed, like Cyrano de Begerac in the film, be able to brag about our unwavering panache throughout life!

Or, if you prefer, how Abraham Maslow put it: "Anybody, under any circumstance whatsoever, can be a psychological success—at least in the sense of doing the best that one can and doing fully what one can—to be himself or herself and to accept the reality of himself or herself."

Not to mention, growth / 'neurogenesis' is good for our health and well-being. See Svoboda (2022) in Wellpower in Further Reading for how brain-cell growth can halt mood disorders or prevent them from emerging. This is significant, given the rising rates of depression and anxiety in the world today.

So that's step five, improving your relationship with willpower. Instead of resigning yourself to the whims of prevailing social-psychological forces (i.e., without willpower), you can learn to see willpower as your *superpower*. Gifting you the ability to set bold goals, knowing that means constructively dealing with all the accompanying growing pains such as tolerating discomfort, recovering from setbacks, delaying gratification, etc.

Accepting it's simply the price to be paid to get to where you want to go and who you aspire to become. Most notably, in finding ways to achieve it, without losing yourself in the process, you will achieve the ultimate reward: finding your true or best self!

Step Six: Retain permission to be human.

In the 2006 film 'Click,' Adam Sandler was given a magical remote control. He could use it to choose to fast-forward, rewind, or pause life. Adam became fixated on 'fast-forwards.' He wanted to know what the future had in store for him and to bypass the drudgery and hard work en route. This succeeded, but he also skipped years of life events in the process, and his life had literally passed him by. The message is we can't spend our lives forever in fast-forward mode. We need to appreciate the ride and not get unduly wrapped up in achieving our goals at the expense of our larger mission or purpose in life.

Undoubtedly, as desirable a quality as ambition is, a flexible attitude is equally deserving. Many people favour spontaneity as much as they value willpower, and as such, they seek a healthy balance between the two. Too much rigidity or time spent on autopilot mode can dehumanise us. It causes us to miss out on profound human experiences, that form the film script of our lives, and that shape our ever-evolving personal identity.

What's more, when we overly rely on 'cool rational' thinking relative to everyday 'hot emotions,' we can start to lose our way in the world. We become like the Tin-Man in the Wizard of Oz, in search of a 'heart.'

The solution is to give yourself, in positive psychologist Tal Ben-Shahar's words, 'permission to be human'. That is to permit yourself small pleasures and mini enjoyments rather than thinking you have to soldier on relentlessly. To also factor in ample time for spontaneous events to happen, since positive emotions like excitement, serendipity, awe, and surprise need space to thrive. It's what makes life meaningful, colourful and memorable.

Whilst a belief in unlimited willpower may overcome mild depletion; it can prove counter-productive if taken too far. A case of when one of our strengths can become our kryptonite. It's not always about living in anticipation of a brighter future, delaying gratification, and dismissing the present. It's important to know when to hold back or stop something. To know when good is good enough, in the overall scheme of things. To accept less than our best when our best is asking too much of us, or puts us at risk of unhealthy perfectionism.

"We are both ants and grasshoppers, and to lose the hot emotional system and live continually dominated by the cool cognitive system in the service of a possible future can become a life story as unsatisfying as its opposite."
- Walter Mischel

It means valuing contentment as much as accomplishment; holding onto future aspirations whilst being grateful for the present; finding success without losing sight of everything that makes life rich and worthwhile.

Above all, ensuring we have sufficient willpower reserves to be at choice; rather than being led by blind ambition and going all out forcefully driving desired change into being. Yes, granting ourselves permission to be human.

Step Seven: Fast Forwards (consulting with your future self).

Willpower is required when a present-oriented system clashes with a future-oriented valuation system. Consulting with your future self then is a novel way of bridging this gap, with present self portraying the doer (i.e., the one who is vulnerable to temptations) and future self the planner (i.e., the one in charge of willpower).

By repeatedly envisioning your future self, you familiarize yourself with its wants, needs, desires, intentions, standards, etc. You might compare it to asking your future self about the likely implications of any intended decision. Present self assumes the collaborative role of supporting future self in advancing their mutual interests. No longer is future self the scapegoat, left to deal with the repercussions of poor choices made by present self.

It's also what healthy, high-functioning brains do best: prediction and self-regulation. Our brains rewind and replay experiences in our minds, plus pause and contemplate the present, in order to make the best possible decision regarding the immediate future. They also favour efficiency, repeating past successful behaviours, as opposed to undertaking any new or different challenge of any magnitude.

However, reality is negotiable. We can learn to better predict the future. We can reject the easy option of simply replicating our past, i.e., what's probable. Instead, we can pursue a sense of what's possible.

Some of you may be familiar with wormholes in quantum physics. Wormholes represent a shortcut between two end points in space-time. We don't actually know they physically exist, but wouldn't it be great mentally if we could Fast Forwards our minds to a future space and time (i.e., a future self perspective)? Equally to be able to zoom back again armed with new insights.

Thereupon not only leaning on past experience, as is the norm, but also drawing from future experience. In other words, a two-way memory system encompassing a past and a future timeline:

'It's a poor sort of memory that only works backwards,' the Queen remarked."
— Lewis Carroll, Through the Looking-Glass and What Alice
Found There

The above quote is from The Queen of Hearts chastising Alice in Wonderland for not comprehending a memory system that works both ways.

Adopting this mental model, Fast Forwards offers a way of knowing where you are headed. Future memories lay the groundwork for fusing your present with the future.

As such, your ability to fast-forward your mind – 'to consult with your future self' - is a seldom mentioned piece of the willpower puzzle. The more continuity you can feel or see between 'you now' and 'future you,' the more likely you are to invest in and prioritise that 'future self'. We all have this image of an 'ideal self', this elaborate construct of who we would like to be. Our natural inclination is to want to live up to this expectation, or else we feel restless and moody.

You can purposefully shape who you become, then. by looking forward in an optimistic way to your aspirations and to whom you need to become in order to attain them.

This is different from the traditional change model. You are not seeking to change who you are as a person based on your current self's state. You are optimising from your future self's perspective, a more advantageous vantage point from which to set and prioritise your life goals. Loosening your hold on your current perspective also opens up your mind to possibility. You become less attached to your current self and more committed to your future self.

New Year resolutions often don't work because we resolve to be what amounts to a totally different person. There's a mental and emotional disconnect... and before January is over, we get found out. By setting up a daily Fast Forwards practice of imagining and rehearsing how you want to BE, you evolve with time into that person. The change process is more incremental than revolutionary, improving the odds of change sticking.

It recognises too that your concept of 'self' is under constant construction and is forever evolving in the direction of your imprinting. Just compare 'past you' – say, you ten years ago - with 'present you.' Now think 'future you' looking ten years ahead. Is it not likely a more mature or advanced version of your 'present self'? I hope so! After all, is life not principally about growth?

The concept of 'future memories' is also not as crazy as it might first appear to you. Athletes have been mastering visualisation skills for years in a variety of sports, from golf to football and athletics. Given the narrow margins in elite level sport these days, it has proven invaluable to some. Memory experts also teach us we can't be certain of the accuracy of our past recollections. We are constantly reconstructing past experiences, meaning it's possible to have false memories! It's why there's great value in being able to 'let go' and in having the capacity to reframe or reinterpret past events in therapy sessions. With this in mind, Lewis Carroll might have been ahead of his time in seeing memory as capable of operating in both directions.

Try it now for yourself. Fast Forwards your current age by 25 years. It's your birthday party, and your best friend is giving a speech. What would you hope they were saying about you? How clear and compelling is your vision? How optimistic are you about your future? Who surrounds you? What did it cost you to get there? What future memory comes to mind for you?!

There's one important final caveat. Enjoy the Fast Forwards process. In reality, there is no perfect blueprint or single, coherent sense of self to be found. Our identity encompasses multiple dimensions of self and is constantly in flux, so there is little point in overdefining or taking ourselves too seriously. The dark side of self-discovery is that we can become arrogant and overly fixated on ourselves. Life has a knack for pruning away at us with its shears until we get over ourselves and accept that life is far bigger than any one of us alone.

Stepping constructively into our future selves' shoes takes humility, curiosity, restraint, empathy, and experimentation – or else we run the risk of missing things. We should freely permit ourselves the psychological flexibility of allowing various versions of our future selves to emerge and develop as the moment dictates. After all, it's only through the shedding of our present self's skin that we grow and morph over time into our 'future self.'

This way, we get to constantly invent ourselves as we go, making our dent on the world, which in turn leaves its mark on us. It's how we advance through life, feeling that we, as individuals, matter and have something to contribute. It's also how we find reserves of willpower we never knew we had.

KEY CHAPTER TAKEAWAYS:

1) Fill your tank and/or fix the leaks. You can't expect to have reserves of willpower if you are running on near-empty (mentally, emotionally, or physically).

2) Those with high willpower have set up their lives in such a way as to apply willpower judiciously – i.e., only when deemed necessary, in service to a bigger YES.

3) The secret behind a bigger YES rests in the strength of our imagination, in being able to *fast forwards* and preview what attractions await us in life - i.e., trusting your future self to be your consultant or mentor.

9. CONCLUSION

We live in the perfect storm for willpower depletion: being bombarded by complex demands and over-committed with good intentions to 'catch up' soon. Nonetheless, we all are blessed with this inner resource that instructs our mind to be at choice as opposed to acting impulsively, automatically, or in response to outer forces.

In that sense, willpower is our superpower:

"Willpower is the strength of mind that your future will be better than the present, with you commanding the power to make it so."

It hands us the keys to freedom, peace-of-mind, well-being, and the capacity to evolve so that we can live our deepest truth, whatever that may be. In the words of George Bernard Shaw, a power that positions us 'to be able to choose the line of greatest (personal) advantage, instead of yielding in the direction of the least resistance.'

It requires a degree of daring to live life on your terms rather than meekly follow the socially acceptable 'default path'. Willpower provides this. It hones our focus, syncs our actions with the bigger picture, reveals our potential, and steers us in the right direction. In doing so, willpower permits us fortitude over regret and growth over conformity - infusing us with the resolve to persevere even when events do not turn out the way we might like.

Not living a life true to you was the top regret in the book, 'The 5 Regrets of the Dying' by Bronnie Ware, as espoused by the sentiment, "I wish I'd had the courage to live a life true to myself (not the life others expected of me)." Regret leaves us with that unfinished feeling of 'what if' or 'if only________.' Perhaps that's why we regret more what we didn't try (and missed out on) than what we did try (and did not succeed in)? Willpower represents our insurance against regret.

So by now, I trust you grasp that willpower matters and have a greater awareness of how best to utilise this potent strength. Get it right, and you will have all the necessary drive, focus, and self-assurance you need to intentionally manifest your desired future. Yes, the future may appear at times uncertain. However, you can get better at entertaining it by having faith in your 'future self' to act as your confidant and mentor.

By matching what you want with whom you aspire to be and living in harmony with that inspired vision, you can bring that future into the present. Most rewarding of all, you bloom into your 'best self' in the process.

There rests the hidden key to willpower: your capacity to Fast Forwards and see what lies ahead, to determine to do what's most favourable for you in the long haul. It not only enables you to live your best life, but it also gets the very best out of you.

Scientific American recently ran the headline: 'Free will is only an illusion if you are, too.' (January 2023). I agree. Willpower is a very real force that grants you the chance to make something of your life (and yourself in the process).

Always remember: Where there's a will, there's a way. Nil desperadum.

10 FURTHER READING

1) Well Power

André, N. and Baumeister, R.F. (November, 2022). Three Pathways Into Chronic Lack of Energy As A Mental Health Complaint. European Journal of Health Psychology. Health Psychology. Vol 0, Issue 0. https://doi.org/10.1027/2512-8442/a000123

Bernecker, K. et al (September, 2017). Implicit Theories About Willpower Predict Subjective Well-Being. Journal of Personality, 85(2):136-150. https://doi.org/10.1111/jopy.12225

Svoboda, E. (August, 2022) Brain-Cell Growth Keeps Mood Disorders At Bay. Nature. https://doi.org/10.1038/d41586-022-02210-z

Wiehler, A. et al (August, 2022). A Neuro-Metabolic Account Of Why Day Long Cognitive Work Alters The Control Of Economic Decisions. Current Biology. Vol 32, Issue 16. https://doi.org/10.1016/j.cub.2022.07.010

2) Who Power

Eckert, M. (December, 2016). Overcome Procrastination: Enhancing Emotion Regulation Skills Reduce Procrastination, Learning and Individual Differences, Vol 52, pages 10-18. https://doi.org/10.1016/j.lindif.2016.10.001

Hampson, S. (December, 2017). Personality and Health. Oxford Research Encyclopedia of Psychology. https://doi.org/10.1093/acrefore/9780190236557.013.121

Hoffer, A & Giddings, L. (October, 2015). Exercising Willpower: Differences In Willpower Depletion Among Athletes And Nonathletes. Contemporary Economic Policy. Vol 34, Issue 3. https://doi.org/10.1111/coep.12150

McCown W. (April, 1989) The Relationship Between Impulsivity, Empathy And Involvement In Twelve Step Self-Help Substance Abuse Treatment Groups. Br J Addict. 84(4):391-3. https://doi.org/10.1111/j.1360-0443.1989.tb00582.x

Schmeichel, B. J., and Vohs, K. (2009). Self-Affirmation And Self-Control: Affirming Core Values Counteracts Ego Depletion. Journal of Personality and Social Psychology, 96(4), 770–782. https://doi.org/10.1037/a0014635

3) Permission to be Human

Bajaj, K. (January, 2023) Routines Are Great, But Spontaneity Is The Key To Brain Expansion. https://www.mindbodygreen.com/articles/why-being-spontaneous-is-key-to-mental-health

Chappell, R.Y. (July, 2017). Willpower Satisficing. Noûs, 53: 251-265. https://doi.org/10.1111/nous.12213

Grubiak K.P. et al (January, 2022), Taking The New Year's Resolution Test Seriously: Eliciting Individuals' Judgements About Self-Control And Spontaneity. Behavioural Public Policy, pp. 1 - 23. https://doi.org/10.1017/bpp.2021.41

Irving, Z. C. et al (2022). The Shower Effect: Mind Wandering Facilitates Creative Incubation During Moderately Engaging Activities. Psychology of Aesthetics, Creativity, and the Arts. https://doi.org/10.1037/aca0000516

Segar, M. (Nov, 2022). It's Time to Unhabit. Am J Health Promot. 36(8):1418-1420. https://doi.org/10.1177/08901171221125326f

4) Why Power

Ainslie, G. (August, 2020). Willpower With And Without Effort. Behav Brain Sci. 44:e30. https://doi.org/10.1017/S0140525X20000357

Audiffren, M. et al (April, 2022). Training Willpower: Reducing Costs and Valuing Effort. Front. Neurosci. 16:699817. https://doi.org/10.3389/fnins.2022.699817

Baumeister, R.F., Vohs, K.D. (August 2007). Self-Regulation, Ego Depletion, and Motivation. Volume1, Issue1. Social and Personality Psychology Compass. https://doi.org/10.1111/j.1751-9004.2007.00001.x

Inzlicht, M. et al (April, 2018) The Effort Paradox: Effort Is Both Costly and Valued Trends. Cogn Sci 22(4): 337–349. https://doi.org/10.1016/j.tics.2018.01.007

Irving, Z.C. et al (August, 2022). Will-Powered: Synchronic Regulation Is The Difference Maker For Self-Control. Cognition, Vol 225, 105154. https://doi.org/10.1016/j.cognition.2022.105154

Quirin, M. et al. (March 2021). Effortless Willpower? The Integrative Self and Self-Determined Goal Pursuit. Front Psychol. Vol 12 https://doi.org/10.3389/fpsyg.2021.653458
Uziel, L. et al, (2021). What Makes People Want More Self-Control: A Duo Of Deficiency And Necessity. Motivation Science, 7(3), 242–251. https://doi.org/10.1037/mot0000213
Woolley, K. and Fishbach, A. (March, 2022) Motivating Personal Growth by Seeking Discomfort. Volume 33, Issue 4. https://doi.org/10.1177/09567976211044685

5) Way Power
Bermúdez, J.P. (February, 2021) The Skill Of Self-Control. Synthese 199, 6251–6273. https://doi.org/10.1007/s11229-021-03068-w
Kirgios, E.L. et al (November, 2020). Teaching Temptation Bundling To Boost Exercise: A Field Experiment, Organizational Behaviour and Human Decision Processes, Vol 161, pages 20-35. https://doi.org/10.1016/j.obhdp.2020.09.003
Lowe, M. R et el. (January, 2018) Evaluation Of Meal Replacements And A Home Food Environment Intervention For Long-Term Weight Loss. The American Journal of Clinical Nutrition. 107 (1) https://doi.org/10.1093/ajcn/nqx005
Sherman, D. K. (November, 2013). Self-Affirmation: Understanding The Effects. Social and Personality Psychology Compass, 7(11), 834–845. https://doi.org/10.1111/spc3.12072

6) Social Power
Davis, A.J. et al (September, 2021) Social Reward And Support Effects On Exercise Experiences And Performance: Evidence From Parkrun. PLoS ONE 16(9): e0256546. https://doi.org/10.1371/journal.pone.0256546
Tunçgenç, B. et al (January, 2023) Social Bonds Are Related To Health Behaviors And Positive Well-Being Globally. Sci Adv.9(2) https://doi.org/10.1126/sciadv.add3715
Yahya J (June, 2021) Breaking Beyond the Borders of the Brain: Self-Control as a Situated Ability. Front. Psychol. https://doi.org/10.3389/fpsyg.2021.617434

7) Willpower

Lamichhane, B. et al (August, 2022). Delay Of Gratification Dissociates Cognitive Control And Valuation Brain Regions In Healthy Young Adults. Neuropsychologia. Vol 173, 108303. https://doi.org/10.1016/j.neuropsychologia.2022.108303

Dobryakova E, + Smith D.V. (September, 2022) Reward Enhances Connectivity Between The Ventral Striatum And The Default Mode Network. NeuroImage, Vol 258, 119398. https://doi.org/10.1016/j.neuroimage.2022.119398

Warren B. (July, 2012) The Top Five Regrets of the Dying: A Life Transformed by the Dearly Departing by Bronnie Ware. Proc (Bayl Univ Med Cent). 25(3):299–300. PMCID: PMC3377309.

ABOUT THE AUTHOR

WellCoach Noel Lyons is a UK based Executive Coach, helping high-performing but time-challenged professionals - worldwide - maximise their *mental* fitness.

Noel holds a 2.1 in Physical Education from Birmingham University, a Masters in Exercise + Health Science from Bristol University, plus professional Coaching qualifications.
Drawing on over 30 years of international work experience, Noel thrives on mixing the latest science with best practise. Founder of WellCoach UK since 2004, Noel has helped guide and inspire countless people from dedicated service professionals to leading entrepreneurs, to sporting elite, and even royalty (including having once supervised a basketball session between Princes William and Harry).

FINDING YOUR BEST
What's the highest Vision you have for yourself?

Finding your BEST means be able to sustain high levels of clarity, focus and confidence. This way, you are more likely to achieve mighty goals and have the health and energy to enjoy their rewards as well. To explore how small shifts can add up to BIG differences in your life, email Noel - mailto: wellcoachnoel@gmail.com - to arrange a free 15 minute "Finding Your Best" coaching call

One Last Thing
Thank you for reading this far.
I do hope you have found this book of value.
Noel